SCARY CASES
in Otolaryngology

SCARY CASES
in Otolaryngology

Michael P. Platt, MSc, FAAOA
Kenneth M. Grundfast, MD, FACS

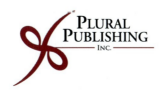

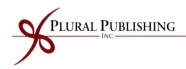

5521 Ruffin Road
San Diego, CA 92123

e-mail: info@pluralpublishing.com
Website: http://www.pluralpublishing.com

Copyright © 2017 by Plural Publishing, Inc.

Typeset in 11/13 Garamond by Flanagan's Publishing Services, Inc.
Printed in Korea by Four Colour Print Group

All rights, including that of translation, reserved. No part of this publication may be reproduced, stored in a retrieval system, or transmitted in any form or by any means, electronic, mechanical, recording, or otherwise, including photocopying, recording, taping, Web distribution, or information storage and retrieval systems without the prior written consent of the publisher.

For permission to use material from this text, contact us by
Telephone: (866) 758-7251
Fax: (888) 758-7255
e-mail: permissions@pluralpublishing.com

Every attempt has been made to contact the copyright holders for material originally printed in another source. If any have been inadvertently overlooked, the publishers will gladly make the necessary arrangements at the first opportunity.

NOTICE TO THE READER
Care has been taken to confirm the accuracy of the indications, procedures, drug dosages, and diagnosis and remediation protocols presented in this book and to ensure that they conform to the practices of the general medical and health services communities. However, the authors, editors, and publisher are not responsible for errors or omissions or for any consequences from application of the information in this book and make no warranty, expressed or implied, with respect to the currency, completeness, or accuracy of the contents of the publication. The diagnostic and remediation protocols and the medications described do not necessarily have specific approval by the Food and Drug administration for use in the disorders and/or diseases and dosages for which they are recommended. Application of this information in a particular situation remains the professional responsibility of the practitioner. Because standards of practice and usage change, it is the responsibility of the practitioner to keep abreast of revised recommendations, dosages, and procedures.

Library of Congress Cataloging-in-Publication Data

Names: Platt, Michael P., editor. | Grundfast, Kenneth, editor.
Title: Scary cases in otolaryngology / [edited by] Michael P. Platt, Kenneth
  M. Grundfast.
Description: San Diego, CA : Plural Publishing, Inc., [2017] | Includes
  bibliographical references.
Identifiers: LCCN 2016027627| ISBN 9781597566544 (alk. paper) | ISBN
  1597566543 (alk. paper)
Subjects: | MESH: Otorhinolaryngologic Diseases | Otorhinolaryngologic
  Surgical Procedures—methods | Otolaryngology | Case Reports
Classification: LCC RF56 | NLM WV 140 | DDC 617.5/1—dc23
LC record available at https://lccn.loc.gov/2016027627

CONTENTS

Foreword: What We Learn From the Imperfect   ix
George J. Annas

Preface: What Is a Scary Case?   xiii
Kenneth M. Grundfast

Acknowledgments   xv

Contributors   xvii

Section 1   AIRWAY   1

Chapter 1   Anesthesia Foreign Body: It's Not Over Until It's Over   3
Daryl Colden and Christopher Jayne

Chapter 2   Airway Foreign Body: Simulation in Action   9
Gi Soo Lee and David W. Roberson

Chapter 3   Tracheostomy: An Unusual Indication   15
Edward J. Reardon

Chapter 4   Airway Fire: Why Are They Called "Laser-Resistant" Tubes?   21
Timothy D. Anderson

Section 2   RISK MANAGEMENT   29

Chapter 5   The Uninsured Patient: Maintaining the Standard of Care   31
Wendy B.R. Stern

Chapter 6   Facial Plastic Surgery: The Case Without End   39
Jeffrey H. Spiegel

Chapter 7   Malingering: An Unusual Stapedectomy Outcome   47
Terry J. Garfinkle

Chapter 8   Four Things to Keep in Mind to Make Those Scary Cases a Little Less Formidable   53
Anthony E. Abeln

Chapter 9   Malpractice Defense From the Expert Witness Perspective   57
R. William Mason

Section 3   MEDICAL ETHICS   63

Chapter 10   Decision-Making Capacity: You Don't Want to Have Surgery, But You Have to Have Surgery   65
Kevin S. Emerick

Chapter 11	Facial Excision: Maintaining Control in the Face of Cancer *Daniel G. Deschler*	73
Chapter 12	Unrelenting Ménière Disease: Ear Surgery in an Only Hearing Ear *Daniel J. Lee and Samuel R. Barber*	85
Chapter 13	Unexpected Lymphoma: The Routine Scary Case *Jerry M. Schreibstein*	97
Chapter 14	Tracheotomy: A Scary Chief Complaint *Bruce R. Gordon*	105

Section 4 NEURAL INJURY — 113

Chapter 15	Orbital Hematoma: In the Public Eye *Ralph Metson and Christopher David Brook*	115
Chapter 16	Facial Nerve Injury: The Service Recovery Paradox *Kimberly A. Russell and Robert W. Dolan*	125
Chapter 17	Encephalocele: An Unexpected Finding *Jonathon Sillman*	131
Chapter 18	Intracranial Extension: A Benign Disease? *Scharukh Jalisi, Avner Aliphas, Samuel J. Rubin, and Kenneth M. Grundfast*	139
Chapter 19	Skull Base Injury: A Scary Harpoon *Ameer T. Shah and Walid I. Dagher*	149
Chapter 20	Brain Herniation: A Delayed Complication *Scharukh Jalisi, Samuel J. Rubin, and Kevin Wu*	159

Section 5 VASCULAR INJURIES — 169

Chapter 21	Aberrant Carotid: A Bloody Myringotomy *Yehia Mohammed Ashry and Dennis S. Poe*	171
Chapter 22	Radiation Therapy for Laryngeal Cancer: "Organ Preservation" *Jonathan C. Simmonds and Elie Rebeiz*	181
Chapter 23	Helicopter Flight: A Scary Post-Tonsillectomy Bleed *Edward F. Caldwell and Hani Ibrahim*	187
Chapter 24	Sentinel Bleed: The Saturday Night Bleeder *Barry J. Benjamin and Namita R. Murthy*	193

Section 6 PROFESSIONALISM — 197

Chapter 25	It Was Not Your Fault! *Charles W. Vaughan*	199

Chapter 26	Tunnel Vision: Too Little . . . Too Late . . . *Scott Finlay and Mark S. Volk*	203
Chapter 27	Chronic Traumatic Encephalopathy: Who Wants to Fight? *Michael P. Platt and Robert A. Stern*	211
Chapter 28	Helping Your Colleague: No Good Deed Goes Unpunished *Aaron R. Dezube, Christopher W. Tsang, and Mark Vecchiotti*	223

FOREWORD

What We Learn From the Imperfect

Surgeon-writer Richard Selzer observes in his *The Doctor Stories* that "doctors write [stories] every day in the charts of patients."[1] Storytelling is integral to the practice of medicine. The patient tells his or her story to the surgeon, who then explains the options available to address the patient's problem. Surgeons often repeat, and restructure, patient stories when consulting with other surgeons. Some storytelling is ritualistic and even superficial. Selzer, after he had retired from surgery to write full time, thought that "looking back, I cannot help but think that my best writing was done in the charts of my patients [because] it was devoid of the vanity of the author . . . and the life at risk was not my own."[1] The stories in this collection draw their power from the drama described in medical charts—but go well beyond the facts and diagnoses to provoke reflection on risk and uncertainty in surgery. They are surgeons' stories about their self-selected "scary" encounters with patients—often focused on a mistake or a bad outcome.

Bad outcomes are inevitable in surgery, as in every human endeavor. *To Err is Human*, the title of a well-known report from the National Academy of Medicine about medical errors, reflects this reality. Measures are contested, but medical errors have recently been ranked as the third leading cause of death in the United States, after heart disease and cancer.[2] Most of the scary cases in this book are based on the personal experiences of an otolaryngologist who is trying to treat a very sick patient, and were initially shared with colleagues at an annual Halloween conference. What makes the encounter "scary"—and Halloween worthy—is usually that the surgeon is worried that his or her actions could result in a bad medical outcome for the patient leading to a bad legal outcome for the surgeon: a malpractice suit. Surgeons often equate "scary" with "I could get sued," and there is almost always a ghost-like character lurking in the background of these stories: the malpractice attorney.

Fear is magnified by ignorance. The most innovative aspect of this collection is the invitation to malpractice lawyers to comment, and to make suggestions of how surgeons can avoid being sued. Perhaps surprisingly, physician-attorney interactions are, at least usually, beneficial to both professions. As one of the first editors of the *New England Journal of Medicine*, Walter Channing, put it more than 150 years ago: "Medicine and law, two of the most diverse callings, may act in perfect harmony, and for the equal benefit of both." Channing also quoted medicolegal expert David Paul Brown who said, "A doctor who knows nothing of law, and a lawyer who knows nothing of medicine, are deficient in essential requisites of their respective professions."[3] I think the judgments of both Channing and Brown remain insightful today, and I also believe that education should begin early.

I have taught law at Boston University School of Medicine for 4 decades. (I also teach health law at the Law School.) Medical students are simultaneously eager to learn and leery of lawyers. Even as first-year medical students, at least some already see lawyers as predators and physicians as prey. Some of this suspicion can be traced to lawyers who advertise for business on television, and give physicians the impression that they are out to get them and are primarily motivated by money. This is partially true, but incomplete. Law supports the practice of medicine, and judges and juries identify with physicians.

There is much to know about the law, but for physicians generally, and surgeons in particular, there are two fundamental legal principles that can make their professional lives less stressful, and they can be easily summarized: Act consistent with the medical standard of care (what a reasonably prudent physician would do in the same or similar circumstances), with your patient's informed consent (including disclosure of the risks and alternatives—and their risks). And, in an emergency, treat first and ask legal questions later. The cases in this volume are written by surgeons who understand the importance of living up to the profession's "standard of care," and of obtaining the patient's informed consent before performing surgery. The case by William Mason illustrates how physicians and lawyers can learn from each other and work constructively together. Mason insightfully and lucidly uses his personal experience as a defendant in a lawsuit (he ultimately prevailed at a jury trial) to learn about the legal system, and to discover the high regard juries and judges have for physicians. Mason accepts an invitation to work with lawyers as an expert reviewer and witness in cases of alleged medical malpractice. He sees his work as an expert witness as rewarding in itself, but also as a service to the medical profession.

The thread running through these stories is fear of medical malpractice litigation, but the prospect of becoming a defendant in a malpractice case is hardly the only reason a clinical encounter can be scary. The encounter can also be scary because it involves a surprising, emergency condition, or simply presents a very complex medical condition that has no simple or safe surgical solution. Specific examples presented include patients with Ménière disease and Munchausen syndrome; and especially unusual cases involving doing surgery on live TV, and having an uninsured patient who cannot afford treatment work at the physician's house in exchange for care. There is even one instance in which the case is scary for the surgeon because his violent patient, a former professional hockey player who had likely taken too many blows to the head in his hockey career, threatens to harm the surgeon and his family. And, of course, from the patient's perspective, head and neck surgery is always scary.

These stories also illustrate how much surgery—and health care in general—has evolved to take informed consent seriously, and to move, slowly but surely, beyond a "culture of silence" to a culture of safety. When mistakes happen, it is now seen as reasonable and ethical to inform the patient and try to make sure similar mistakes don't happen again. Open discussion of mistakes is critical to the patient safety movement. In one particularly bizarre story, Mark Volk recalls an incident from 1984 when he was a first-year surgical resident. Late at night a medical resident paged him to start an arterial line on a 63-year-old patient. Medical residents had been trying unsuccessfully for almost an hour to place the line. Volk began his attempt by telling the patient, "I'm Dr. Volk, and I'm going to try and see if I can place this line in your wrist." He could not, so he moved to the femoral artery. No pulse. He then noticed, among other things, that the patient's pupils were fixed and dilated, and realized that the patient had likely been dead for some time. Volk turned to the residents and nurses in the room and declared: "You can't get an art line because he doesn't have a radial pulse and he doesn't have a radial pulse because he's DEAD!" and walked out. Volk follows his almost perfect Halloween story by explaining how it could have happened (by being fixated on one particular task), and how he would react much differently today because the culture of medicine has changed: quality and safety have moved to the forefront, and "a root-cause analysis would have been convened."

At the 2012 Scary Cases conference, I spoke about "standard of care" and took advantage of the invitation to tell my own "old time medicine" story, this time from the patient's viewpoint. My story was from 1965, when I was a college student. I was waiting in one of about 50 cubicles in a large room at a local hospital when I overheard part of a conversation in the next cubicle. I couldn't make it out, and apparently neither could the patient. The physician repeated it, slowly and very loudly: "You have a tumor in your ear, but it's ALL RIGHT because the doctor can't see you for SIX MONTHS." Whether or not this was scary to the patient—it was certainly scary to me and obviously did not reflect either good standard of care or informed consent, to say nothing of patient confidentiality. Practice really has changed, and not just because of the Health Insurance Portability and Accountability Act (HIPAA) and fear of malpractice lawsuits for failure to diagnose cancer while it may be treatable.

Halloween is celebrated by wearing costumes and trying to scare ourselves and others. Medicine is symbolized by a costume as well: a white coat. The purpose of the white coat is the opposite of the Halloween costume: to comfort and reassure patients who may be facing major life-changing conditions that the physician will put the patient's interests first, and is sworn to "do no harm." As scary as most of them are, I found the stories in this book strangely comforting. This is because, I think, they expose and reflect a practice of surgery, at least of otolaryngology, that is patient centered and populated by surgeons who take both the standard of care and the patient's informed consent seriously. From their 1860 perspective, Walter Channing and David Paul Brown might also add that otolaryngologists inviting lawyers to their Scary Cases conferences can provide "equal benefit to both."

—George J. Annas, JD, MPH
Warren Distinguished Professor and Director
Center for Health Law, Ethics and Human Rights
Boston University School of Public Health

REFERENCES

1. Richard Selzer, The Doctors Stories. New York: Picador; 1998:16.
2. Makary M, Daniel M. Medical error: The third leading cause of death in the US. *BMJ* 2016;353:2139.
3. Annas GJ. Doctors, patients, and lawyers: Two centuries of health law. *N Engl J Med* 2012;367:445-450.

PREFACE

What Is a Scary Case?

Physicians, especially surgeons, like to get good results. But, things do not always go well. There was a time when physicians were reluctant to discuss with others less than optimal outcomes of treatments provided for patients. A century ago in 1916, a leap forward occurred in the way that doctors discuss with each other outcomes from patient care when Dr. Ernest Codman introduced at the Massachusetts General Hospital the concept of having morbidity and mortality conferences. For the past hundred years, hospital-based morbidity and mortality conferences have became the standard method utilized by physicians to analyze problems that have occurred with patient care and to share information with each other.

The *Scary Cases* conferences that began on Halloween Day in Boston in 2010 represent another leap forward in the way that physicians exchange information about what has occurred in case management. The Scary Cases conferences have brought together academic physicians, community-based physicians, nonphysician providers, nurses, attorneys, specialists in risk management, and others who focus in a collegial way on errors, near-miss cases, and frightening situations in the management of patients with disorders affecting the head and neck. Somewhat ironically, even though the cases presented primarily are complicated involving actual untoward outcomes or risk of untoward outcomes, discussion about the cases is characterized by mutual respect, empathy, and candor. Presenters usually have tailored their PowerPoint presentations to have a Halloween theme, and some have even worn Halloween costumes while giving their presentations. This may seem incongruous, but, surprisingly, the Halloween theme and the focus on scariness has engendered a collegiality that encourages the presenters and the meeting attendees to share their individual experiences in way that makes the meeting highly informative and extraordinarily valuable.

While reading the cases in this book is not the same as sitting in the audience on Halloween Day listening to a world-renowned otolaryngologist dressed as a Frankenstein monster present a case, reading the cases does provide pithy insights about what can go wrong in the practice of otolaryngology-head and neck surgery along with information about how to avoid trouble and how to get out of trouble. The stylized way in which the cases are written assures that the reader can acquire useful information from the description of each scary case. Life can be scary, the practice of otolaryngology can be scary—the key to success in life and in otolaryngology is to be prepared for whatever happens, not letting fear cloud judgment, and to strive always to do what is right.

—Kenneth M. Grundfast

ACKNOWLEDGMENTS

Scary Cases would only be an idea without the generous contributions of the many clinicians and patients who shared their scary experiences with us. It takes courage to expose our fears and perhaps shortcomings for the benefit of others to learn how to avoid or manage these scary situations. I dedicate this book to my mentors who have provided me with unlimited guidance and support, including Kenneth Grundfast, MD, Ralph Metson, MD, Steven Parnes, MD, Terrence Sweeney, PhD, and Howard Platt, MD.

—*MPP*

I dedicate this book to my mentors M. Stuart Strong, Charles W. Vaughan, Loring W. Pratt, to my lovely wife Ruthanne, and to all otolaryngologists who earnestly strive every day to help their patients even when confronted with scary situations. And, I want to let everyone know that working with Mike Platt on this book and the Scary Cases meetings has been fun, not scary.

—*KMG*

CONTRIBUTORS

Anthony E. Abeln, JD
Partner
Morrison Mahoney LLP
Instructor in Legal Research and Writing
New England Law, Boston
Boston, Massachusetts
Chapter 8

Avner Aliphas, MD
Assistant Professor
Department of Otolaryngology
Boston University School of Medicine
Boston, Massachusetts
Chapter 18

Timothy D. Anderson, MD
Director, Voice and Swallowing
Lahey Clinic
Burlington, Massachusetts
Chapter 4

Yehia Mohammed Ashry, MSc
Department of Otorhinolaryngology
Suez Canal University
Department of Otolaryngology and Communications Enhancement
Boston Children's Hospital
Boston, Massachusetts
Chapter 21

Samuel R. Barber, MS
Research Fellow
Massachusetts Eye and Ear Infirmary
Eaton-Peabody Laboratories
Boston, Massachusetts
Chapter 12

Barry J. Benjamin, MD
Senior Surgeon
Massachusetts Eye and Ear Infirmary
Boston, Massachusetts
Chapter 24

Christopher David Brook, MD
Assistant Professor
Department of Otolaryngology
Boston University School of Medicine
Boston, Massachusetts
Chapter 15

Edward F. Caldwell, MD, FACS
President
Cape Cod ENT Specialists
Cape Cod, Massachusetts
Chapter 23

Daryl Colden, MD
Chief of Surgery
Anna Jaques Hospital
Associate Surgeon in Otolaryngology
Massachusetts Eye and Ear Infirmary
Clinical Instructor in Otology and Laryngology
Harvard Medical School
Boston, Massachusetts
Chapter 1

Walid I. Dagher, MD
ENT Specialists
Boston, Massachusetts
Chapter 19

Daniel G. Deschler, MD, FACS
Vice Chair for Academic Affairs
Director, Norman Knight Hyperbaric Medicine Center
Massachusetts Eye and Ear Infirmary

Professor
Department of Otology and Laryngology
Harvard Medical School
Boston, Massachusetts
Chapter 11

Aaron R. Dezube, MD
Tufts Medical Center
Boston, Massachusetts
Chapter 28

Robert W. Dolan, MD
Chair
Department of Otolaryngology-Head and Neck Surgery
Lahey Health
Burlington, Massachusetts
Chapter 16

Kevin S. Emerick, MD
Assistant Professor
Harvard Medical School
Massachusetts Eye and Ear Infirmary
Boston, Massachusetts
Chapter 10

Scott Finlay, MD
Resident
Department of Otolaryngology-Head and Neck Surgery
Boston Medical Center
Boston, Massachusetts
Chapter 26

Terry J. Garfinkle, MD, MBA, FACS
Chief Medical Officer
Partners Community Physicians Organization
Partners Health Care
Assistant Clinical Professor of Otolaryngology
Harvard Medical School
Massachusetts Eye and Ear Infirmary
Boston, Massachusetts
Chapter 7

Bruce R. Gordon, MA, MD, FACS
Otolaryngology Chief
Cape Cod Hospital
Associate Staff
Massachusetts Eye and Ear Infirmary
Instructor, Laryngology and Otology
Harvard Medical School
Boston, Massachusetts
Chapter 14

Kenneth M. Grundfast, MD, FACS
Professor and Chair
Department of Otolaryngology-Head and Neck Surgery
Assistant Dean
Office of Student Affairs
Boston University School of Medicine
Boston, Massachusetts
Chapter 18

Hani Ibrahim, MD, FACS
Massachusetts Eye and Ear Infirmary
Instructor in Otology and Laryngology
Harvard Medical School
Boston, Massachusetts
Chapter 23

Scharukh Jalisi, MD, MA, FACS
Director, Head and Neck Surgical Oncology
Head and Neck Cancer Center of Excellence
Department of Otolaryngology-Head and Neck Surgery
Boston University
Boston, Massachusetts
Chapters 18 and 20

Christopher Jayne, BA
College of the Holy Cross
Worcester, Massachusetts
Chapter 1

Gi Soo Lee, MD, EdM
Associate in Otolaryngology
Boston Children's Hospital
Instructor
Department of Otology and
 Laryngology
Harvard Medical School
Boston, Massachusetts
Chapter 2

Daniel J. Lee, MD, FACS
Director, Pediatric Ear, Hearing and
 Balance Center
Massachusetts Eye and Ear
 Infirmary
Associate Professor
Department of Otology and
 Laryngology
Harvard Medical School
Boston, Massachusetts
Chapter 12

R. William Mason, MD
Boston ENT Associates
Clinical Assistant Professor
Boston University School of Medicine
Boston, Massachusetts
Chapter 9

Ralph Metson, MD
Professor
Department of Otolaryngology
Harvard Medical School
Boston, Massachusetts
Chapter 15

Namita R. Murthy, MD
Department of Otolaryngology-
 Head and Neck Surgery
Boston University Medical Center
Boston, Massachusetts
Chapter 24

Michael P. Platt, MSc, FAAOA
Associate Professor
Residency Director
Department of Otolaryngology-
 Head and Neck Surgery
Boston University School of
 Medicine
Boston, Massachusetts
Chapter 27

Dennis S. Poe, MD, PhD
Department of Otolaryngology and
 Communications Enhancement
Boston Children's Hospital
Department of Otolaryngology
Harvard Medical School
Boston, Massachusetts
Chapter 21

Edward J. Reardon, MD, FACS
Assistant Clinical Professor
Otology and Laryngology
Harvard Medical School
Massachusetts Eye and Ear
 Infirmary
Chief of Surgery
Beth Israel Deaconess Milton
 Hospital
Boston, Massachusetts
Chapter 3

Elie Rebeiz, MD
Professor and Chair
Otolaryngology-Head and Neck
 Surgery
Tufts Medical Center
Boston, Massachusetts
Chapter 22

**David W. Roberson, MD, FACS,
FRCS**
Associate Professor
Harvard Medical School
Associate in Otolaryngology
Boston Children's Hospital
Boston, Massachusetts
Chapter 2

Samuel J. Rubin, BA
Medical Student
Boston University School of Medicine
Boston, Massachusetts
Chapters 18 and 20

Kimberly A. Russell, MD
Department of Otolaryngology
Boston University Medical Center
Boston, Massachusetts
Chapter 16

Jerry M. Schreibstein, MD, FACS
Ear, Nose and Throat Surgeons of
 Western New England LLC
Assistant Clinical Professor
Otolaryngology-Head and Neck
 Surgery
Tufts University School of Medicine
Springfield, Massachusetts
Chapter 13

Ameer T. Shah, MD
Resident Physician
Department of Otolaryngology-
 Head and Neck Surgery
Tufts Medical Center
Boston, Massachusetts
Chapter 19

Jonathon Sillman, MD, FACS
Assistant Professor
Tufts Department of Otolaryngology
Neurotology, Otology, Skull Base
 Surgery
Boston, Massachusetts
Chapter 17

Jonathan C. Simmonds, MD
Clinical Associate
Department of Otolaryngology-
 Head and Neck Surgery
Tufts Medical Center
Boston, Massachusetts
Chapter 22

Jeffrey H. Spiegel, MD, FACS
Professor and Chief
Facial Plastic and Reconstructive
 Surgery
Department of Otolaryngology-
 Head and Neck Surgery
Boston University School of Medicine
Director, Advanced Facial Aesthetics
Chestnut Hill, Massachusetts
Chapter 6

Wendy B.R. Stern, MD
Southcoast Hospital Group
Dartmouth, Massachusetts
Chapter 5

Robert A. Stern, PhD
Professor of Neurology,
 Neurosurgery, and Anatomy and
 Neurobiology
Director, BU Alzheimer's Disease
 and CTE Center Clinical Care
Boston University School of Medicine
Boston, Massachusetts
Chapter 27

Christopher W. Tsang, MD
Resident Physician
Department of Otolaryngology-
 Head and Neck Surgery
Tufts Medical Center
Boston, Massachusetts
Chapter 28

Charles W. Vaughan, MD
Boston University School of
 Medicine
Boston, Massachusetts
Chapter 25

Mark Vecchiotti, MD
Department of Otolaryngology-
 Head and Neck Surgery
Chief, Division of Pediatric
 Otolaryngology

Director, Pediatric Cochlear Implant Program
Assistant Professor Otolaryngology
Assistant Professor Pediatrics
Floating Hospital for Children at Tufts Medical Center
Boston, Massachusetts
Chapter 28

Mark S. Volk, MD, DMD
Associate in Otolaryngology
Department of Otolaryngology and Communication Disorders
Boston Children's Hospital
Boston, Massachusetts
Chapter 26

Kevin Wu, BS
Boston University School of Medicine
MD Candidate 2017
Boston, Massachusetts
Chapter 20

SECTION 1

Airway

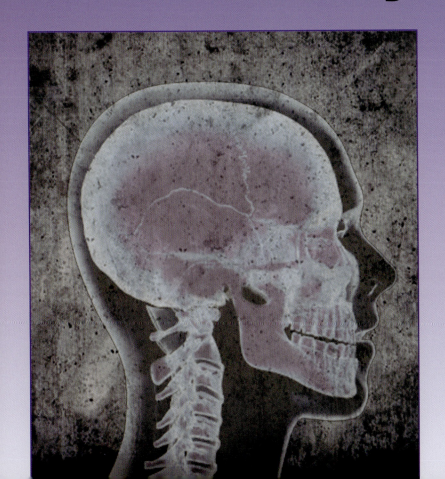

CHAPTER 1

Anesthesia Foreign Body

It's Not Over Until It's Over

Daryl Colden
Christopher Jayne

THE CASE

A 34-year-old man with chronic sinonasal symptoms presented to the otolaryngology clinic. The patient complained of long-standing nasal congestion and trouble breathing through his nose. His symptoms had been present for 5 years and were unimproved with over-the-counter antihistamines and intranasal corticosteroids. His past history was significant for prior nasal trauma. Otherwise his past medical and family history were unremarkable.

Examination of the head and neck revealed a significant nasal septal deviation from the left to right, with approximately 80% obstruction of the nasal passages. There was concomitant bilateral inferior turbinate hypertrophy. Since the patient was symptomatic and not responsive to medical management, he was offered surgical intervention consisting of a septoplasty with an inferior turbinate reduction to be performed under general anesthesia. The patient was agreeable to this surgical plan, and informed consents were obtained. The surgical date was scheduled.

A ROUTINE SURGERY

A standard septoplasty and turbinate reduction using coblation technique were performed under general anesthesia. The patient was intubated without difficulty, and the surgical procedure lasting 50 minutes was uneventful. As my usual routine, silastic nasal splints were sutured to the septum and bilateral Merocel nasal packs were inserted into the nasal cavity to help with hemostasis and improve septal healing. As a resident, I was taught to tie the Merocel nasal packs together across the nasal columella to prevent aspiration. Many words of advice from my mentors came from surgeons who learned the hard way, including aspiration of nasal packs requiring bronchoscopy for removal.

IT'S NOT OVER UNTIL IT'S OVER

At this juncture, the procedure was turned over to the anesthesia team for extubation. I returned to the surgical lounge in order to write postoperative orders and dictate the operative report. Just as I began dictating, the operating room nurse rushed into the lounge stating that the patient was in respiratory distress and had aspirated one of the nasal packs!

I sprinted into the operating room to find the patient upright, unable to speak, and with both of his hands over his neck making the "universal choking sign." The anesthesiologist wasted no time in expressing his displeasure toward me, accusing that the patient had aspirated one of the nasal packs.

I quickly began to evaluate the patient. Evaluation of the nasal cavities revealed both Merocel nasal packs were still tied together and sitting in good position. To be certain, I pulled the two Merocel packs tied together out of the nose. In disbelief, the anesthesiologist noted that there was no improvement in the patient's condition and the patient continued to be in respiratory distress. The surgeon and anesthesiologist looked at each other with concern, both thinking "What's next?" The patient became cyanotic and his oxygen saturation levels started to plummet. I ordered a nurse to prepare the tracheostomy kit while the anesthesiologist began to deliver blow-by oxygen and IV fluids.

GETTING SCARIER

With both physicians unsure of the next step, the surgeon requested that the anesthesiologist administer sedation in order to better evaluate the airway. Sedation of a patient in respiratory distress is often not used, but with a rapidly declining respiratory status and signs of airway obstruction, I needed to be able to evaluate the airway. The anesthesiologist's laryngoscope with a Mack blade was placed and a white foreign body was noted emanating from between the vocal folds. The foreign body was sitting in the larynx—half above the vocal folds and half below the cords. Using Magill forceps, I was able to quickly remove the foreign body. Consequently, the patient was reintubated by the anesthesiologist and slowly extubated. A postoperative chest x-ray was obtained and demonstrated atelectasis but no pneumothorax or signs of pulmonary edema. The patient was treated with IV Unasyn for possible aspiration and he was monitored overnight for possible aspiration pneumonia. He was discharged the following day without any sequelae other than a very sore throat.

WHAT HAPPENED?

The mysterious foreign body that was removed from between the patient's vocal folds was a "fabricated" bite block (Figure 1–1). The bite block consisted of a small rolled-up gauze

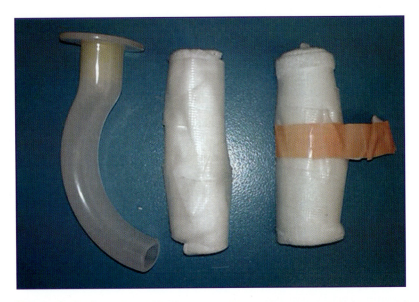

Figure 1–1. Examples of bite blocks used by anesthesiologists during general anesthesia. The variable size, omission from surgical counts, and lack of radiological markings make hand-made bite blocks a potential airway foreign body.

that was taped together. This was originally placed by one anesthesiologist at the beginning of surgery upon intubation. About halfway through the surgical case, a second anesthesiologist relieved the first anesthesiologist and proceeded to finish the surgical case. The bite block most likely had become displaced between the start of the surgical case and the second anesthesiologist taking over. The second anesthesiologist did not know that there was a bite block and would not have been aware that it had become displaced from its original location.

THIS CASE WAS SCARY BECAUSE

There is an old adage: "The lesser the indication, the greater the complication." While the patient certainly fulfilled all of the criteria for elective surgery for quality of life symptoms, the margin for complications is much more narrow in such a surgery compared to a procedure for a life-threatening diagnosis such as head and neck cancer. This patient was a strong, healthy man who was expected to have a favorable outcome from his nasal surgery. The potential for a devastating outcome was present with his airway obstruction.

The situational circumstances of being emergently called back into the room are scary because of the unknown. Surgeons generally are good at maintaining control in the operating room and such an unexpected scenario removes all control from the surgeon. Additionally, the anesthesiologist's accusations that I lost a nasal pack contributed to my fear that I was responsible for the deterioration in my patient's condition. It was ironic that it was his foreign body that caused the airway obstruction.

WHAT I LEARNED FROM THIS CASE

The moral of the story is: It's not over until it's over. One of the most routine ear, nose, throat (ENT) cases performed on an extremely healthy patient almost resulted in a terrible adverse event after the surgeon assumed the case was over. This case is illustrative of many aspects of risk management that the surgeon may assume that he or she is actually a part of. First, although the adverse event occurred mostly due to an error on the part of anesthesiology, the surgeon plays a major role in the recognition of the error and in helping to correct it. The importance of staying calm, acting quickly, and working collaboratively with the surgical team was likely the critical factor in this patient surviving.

In performing a root-cause analysis, there are many areas whereby the risk of this foreign body aspiration could have been avoided. First, the anesthesiologists created their own bite block rather than use the industry-made type. The makeshift bite block was much smaller than the industry-bought type, and therefore more likely to be aspirated and could be lodged between the vocal cords. Second, the bite block was never "counted" or noted. The surgical process these days takes great lengths to make sure everything that the surgeon uses during a procedure is counted and this process mitigates the possibility of a retained foreign body. Why not do the same for anesthesiology? Last, one could argue that during shift changes, there could be greater likelihood of errors as not every piece of critical information can be relayed from one anesthesiology provider to another. An operative case with a short duration, such as a septoplasty/inferior turbinate reduction, should ideally have the same anesthesiology provider present for the duration of the case.

CHAPTER 2

Airway Foreign Body

Simulation in Action

Gi Soo Lee
David W. Roberson

THE CASE

A 13-month-old, otherwise healthy boy was transferred to our emergency department from an outside hospital where he had been evaluated for a persistent wheeze that worsened over the prior 2 days. Parents denied any other acute symptoms consistent with an upper respiratory infection. However, they had noted this wheeze for the past 6 months after a possible aspiration event at home. A chest x-ray revealed a U-shaped metallic object in the left hemithorax within the left main-stem bronchus (Figure 2–1). The patient was transferred for airway endoscopy and foreign body removal. Physical examination revealed a healthy infant without airway distress or increased

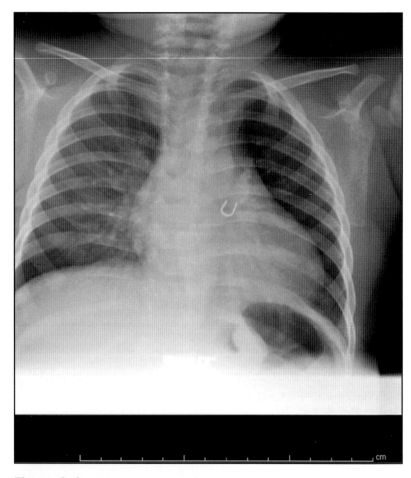

Figure 2–1. Chest x-ray revealed a U-shaped metallic object in the left hemithorax within the left main-stem bronchus.

work of breathing. His oxygen saturation was 94% to 95% on room air, and there were asymmetric breath sounds on auscultation. A subtle wheeze was noted in his left chest. With a diagnosis of an airway foreign body, he was admitted in preparation for the operative procedure.

The patient was taken to the operating room for direct laryngoscopy, rigid tracheobronchoscopy, and removal of the metallic object. A 3.7-mm ventilating bronchoscope was used to identify the foreign body in the distal left mainstem bronchus at the takeoff of the secondary bronchi. It was a construction staple, and the sharp points of the fastener were partially embedded in the bronchial wall. The lumen of the bronchus was narrower than the width of the staple, resulting in the bronchial wall partially conforming around the body of the staple. There was minimal granulation and no purulence in the immediately surrounding region.

It was immediately evident that removal was going to be far more complicated and riskier than originally anticipated given the orientation of the staple within the bronchial wall. Would the bronchus avulse? What if there was profuse bleeding? What if there was a pneumothorax? What if it would *not* come out? The patient was breathing spontaneously under the inhaled anesthetic, and, in reality, was medically stable from a breathing perspective. Given these considerations, we elected to leave the staple in place without disrupting it, awaken the patient, and devise a more structured plan prior to returning to the operating suite. He was sent back to the floor in stable condition.

It was clear to us that we would only get one chance at grasping and removing the object. To better understand what we were going to deal with, we were going to have to practice removing the object prior to actually doing so. Where do we grasp the object, and with which instrument? How would we dislodge the staple points with minimal damage to the bronchial wall? Would it be a straight pull, or would we have to rotate the staple? And so forth.

We needed to build a model to answer these questions.

As we confirmed that the foreign body was a construction staple, we went to a local hardware store and bought several boxes of construction staples of varying sizes and shapes. Using the chest x-ray, we determined it to be an 11-mm steel staple. I opened several endotracheal tubes, again of varying sizes. We were able to slide a staple into a 6-0 ETT and orient it similarly to what we saw in situ; we even embedded the staple points into the ETT wall (Figure 2–2). Then, for the next few hours, I practiced removing the staple from the ETT repeatedly. By trial and error, we discovered that we could grasp the staple near one of the bends with an alligator-shaped forceps and rotate the staple points out of the wall with minimal traction. I then focused on this maneuver several dozen times before feeling reasonably comfortable; the endoscopic video equipment was employed during this practice session to simulate actual removal.

The patient was brought back to the operating room 2 days later, after 48 hours of IV dexamethasone. We had consulted thoracic surgery, and their service was present in the room to assist with any complications that might arise from the procedure. Again, under spontaneous ventilation, we performed our rigid bronchoscopy and encountered the staple. The preoperative steroids had helped clear the small amount of granulation and inflammation in the area. The alligator-tipped optical foreign body forcep was introduced into the bronchoscope. The staple was gently grasped as during our practice session. Then, with the gentlest of tugs . . .

. . . the staple points rolled into the bronchial lumen. The staple was removed from the airway in one smooth maneuver. Success! For the following minute, the room was completely silent as everyone had their eyes glued on the vitals monitor and the anesthesia team to see if anything changed hemodynamically or with oxygenation. Nothing. We ultimately reintroduced the bronchoscopy to inspect the left bronchus—there

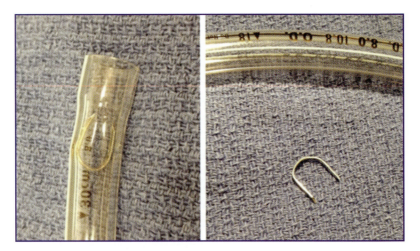

Figure 2–2. We were able to rotate and slide a staple into an endotracheal tube so that it could be removed without damaging the tracheal walls.

was no bleeding, and the secondary bronchi were patent and appeared healthy. We obtained two portable chest x-rays, once in the operating suite, and once an hour later in the recovery room. The patient was discharged the following day.

THIS CASE WAS SCARY BECAUSE

This case was scary, not for what actually happened, but for what *could* have happened had we not been prepared. The metallic foreign body was embedded, and we had no idea whether it was embedded superficially or deeply, or what was on the other side of the wall, whether the lung would collapse upon removal, or how much collateral damage would be caused by extracting the object. The object looked too large to have even been aspirated in the first place. If we presume that the object had been ingested 6 months prior (as the family had suggested), would the tissue be injured or scarred, making the removal complicated? It was the array of potential negative outcomes from removal that made this a scary case.

WHAT I LEARNED FROM THIS CASE

There were several key learning points from this case. First, I learned that, under certain unique circumstances, it is acceptable to *not* complete a procedure. In this case, to leave a foreign body in the airway after we had it in plain sight. The tissues in the region of the staple, in fact, appeared very healthy. Additionally, the patient had been stable with this aspirated object for quite some time. However, because we did not have a better understanding of the object itself (and its relationship to the bronchus), and we were *not* prepared to address any potential complications, we could not comfortably or safely proceed with a risk/benefit balance in our favor. As such, the safer management plan was to terminate the procedure, reassess the situation, make a better plan, and then reattempt.

Second, I learned of the utility of surgical simulation and the effectiveness of deliberate practice in tackling specific surgical problems. We built a specific left main-stem bronchus simulator to help solve our surgical puzzle. Once we had a better understanding of the problem, we could then focus on the actual technique of removing the staple. *Deliberate practice*, a highly structured activity with the specific goal of improving performance, is what a violinist does to master a particular phrase of music, or what a golfer does to perfect a specific sand shot. It involves repetition of a task while actively engaged, and to receive immediate feedback that is used to improve the next iteration of the task. Our simulator allowed us to repeatedly practice removing the staple, and allowed us to finely tune the maneuver with each repetition until we had what we thought would be best for the actual procedure.

Third, I learned the importance of thorough planning and preparation when attempting a deceptively simple yet potentially complex procedure. Discussions with senior colleagues within my department, consultations by other services such as thoracic surgery and radiology, and, perhaps most importantly, discussions with the patient's family were paramount to maximizing the chance of a successful procedure, and to best prepare everyone for a potentially unsuccessful one.

CHAPTER 3

Tracheostomy

An Unusual Indication

Edward J. Reardon

THE CASE

One of the scariest events I have experienced as an otolaryngologist occurred over 30 years ago on a Friday evening at a community hospital 9 miles from Boston. Around 7:30 PM, I was called by the emergency room attending that he was seeing a 16-year-old adolescent girl who was complaining of a moderate sore throat for a few days with a low-grade fever, and she was mildly dehydrated. She had no previous history of tonsillitis, and her only other medical issue was the recent development of asthma. Her physical examination was described as a teenager sitting in bed with normal vital signs except for a low-grade fever. The emergency department physician stated that her pharyngeal examination revealed slightly enlarged tonsils with erythema, no trismus, and minimal adenopathy. Her white blood cell (WBC) count was in the range of 10,000, and the test for mononucleosis was pending. With her dysphagia and mild dehydration, we decided to admit her overnight and to treat her with IV fluids, antibiotics, and steroids. It was a routine case of tonsillitis that I did not need to see as an emergency, until . . .

Three hours later, I was called by the nursing supervisor to come right in as my patient was having progressive agitation and difficulty breathing. My immediate thought was that she had epiglottitis and I asked that anesthesia and the operating room team be called as I headed for the hospital, which was only a few minutes away from my home. When I arrived, I found her in an inpatient floor room on the third floor. She was diaphoretic with inspiratory and expiratory stridor with chest retractions!

The nursing staff had the code cart in the room, and I asked for a headlight and a tracheotomy set. As this was a number of years ago, we did not have O_2 monitors, and I did not carry a flexible laryngoscope in my consult case. I also asked that the emergency room physician come up to help me, and by the time he and the equipment arrived, she seemed to be getting weaker. Still thinking this was epiglottitis, I did not want to trigger complete laryngeal closure by trying to examine her throat and proceeded to do a Jackson 2-slash tracheotomy. I was able to secure the airway without difficulty in this thin, young woman with favorable neck anatomy.

GETTING SCARIER

After the airway was secured and my pulse had slowed down, I called her mother and described what had happened. I was given permission to take her to the operating room to revise the tracheotomy site once anesthesia and the operating room team had arrived. A short time later, I did revise the emergency tracheotomy site to an opening lower in the trachea. My next step was to do a laryngoscopy while she was asleep to obtain cultures and to evaluate the larynx. I was surprised to find a normal larynx. What happened?

My next surprise came a few minutes later when I again called her mother to let her know that surgery was over and that her daughter was stable. I conveyed the findings of a normal larynx and her mother thanked me. She also stated she would be in to see her daughter in the morning, which was a rather bizarre response to a child having gone through a life-threatening experience.

The next morning, I called the pulmonary physician who had recently evaluated this patient for asthma, and he reported that his evaluation for asthma revealed many inconsistencies. Putting everything together, we felt that this was an extreme manifestation of a psychogenic disorder. After discussions with her pediatrician, who knew this family for a long time, this young woman was referred for psychotherapy.

WHAT HAPPENED?

On my way to the hospital that night, I remember thinking that everything had happened so rapidly that the etiology must have been epiglottitis. I also felt that had I examined her earlier that night, this emergency could have been avoided. When I arrived in the hospital room and saw that she was so stridulous and barely moving air, I realized immediately that I was by myself and that I was facing a life-threatening situation with a young woman who could die from airway obstruction. Fortunately, the emergency tracheotomy went well. Although I regretted doing a tracheotomy that was not needed, at the time, my assessment was of impending airway obstruction, hypoxia, and death, and as otolaryngologists we have the expertise and training to prevent such as disaster.

Three months later, in June 1983, an article appeared in the *New England Journal of Medicine* (*NEJM*), "Vocal-Cord Dysfunction Presenting as Asthma" describing a series of five patients with a functional disorder of the vocal cords that mimicked bronchial asthma.[1] During the episodes, each had almost complete adduction of the true vocal cords, the glottis was closed to a small chink and the arytenoids maintained a lateral position during both inspiration and expiration.

Psychologic testing of these patients was consistent with a conversion disorder and they did well with both psychotherapy and speech therapy. They concluded that if a diagnosis can be established, intubation or tracheotomy could be avoided!

One year earlier, Kellman described three patients with stridor caused by paradoxical vocal cord motion.[2] Subsequently, there have been a number of papers in the pediatric, pulmonary, and psychiatry literature describing this entity.[3-5] In the workup of this disorder, consideration has to be given to asthma, gastroesophageal reflux, allergy, infectious diseases, laryngeal irritants, and neurologic and psychiatric conditions. The gold standard for making the diagnosis of paradoxical vocal cord disorder (PVD) is flexible laryngoscopy during an attack. Examinations and pulmonary function tests are normal when the patient is not symptomatic.

More recently, paradoxical vocal fold motion disorder has been diagnosed in high-performance athletes who can greatly benefit from speech therapy and biofeedback.[6,7] Often, long-term corticosteroids can be discontinued and acute episodes can be broken with heliox, which is a mixture of 80% helium and 20% oxygen.

For a few years after this truly scary episode, both my pulmonary colleague and I would occasionally receive emergency room calls from anxious physicians seeing our patient in acute respiratory distress who already had a tracheotomy scar on her neck. It often took a good deal of trust for them to take our advice that she did not need intervention and could be treated supportively. Ultimately, with a combination of psychotherapy and speech therapy, we did not hear of any further emergency room visits and she did benefit from a plastic repair of her tracheotomy scar. Ever since I read the *NEJM* article a few months after the event, I have been on the lookout for articles about paradoxical vocal fold motion disorders including the recent literature on finding this condition in high-performance athletes.

ASK THE EXPERT: Anthony Abeln, JD

Otolaryngologists are taught: "If you think about doing a tracheostomy, it is never wrong to do it."

In general, when one thinks of what the "standard of care" is in a medical malpractice action, the standard is what the *average provider* would do in the doctor's field under the circumstances (with some variation across jurisdictions). That being said, the *judgment* of the physician is a critical factor in the determination of liability. Did the doctor use his or her best judgment when faced with the circumstances of the case?

Imagine the quantum of liability related to tracheostomy? It reaches across two forms. One was where the tracheostomy was performed but later deemed unnecessary because the underlying condition was resolving. On the other end, a physician may have elected not to perform a tracheostomy, and the allegation arises that choice led to a catastrophic result. What is the doctor to do? Damned if I do; damned if I don't . . .

At its crux, if relying on his or her best judgement under the circumstances, the decision is not the wrong one even if the outcome is not ideal. The challenge of the practice of medicine in the era of the medical malpractice lawsuit is the practice of medicine by retrospect-o-scope. If the circumstances make a tracheostomy a procedure that is medically appropriate, and you consider not doing it—why? If it is not medically appropriate and you consider doing it—why? Using your best judgment will often lead you to the correct result.

REFERENCES

1. Christopher KL, Wood RP 2nd, Eckert RC, Blager FB, Raney RA, Souhrada JR. Vocal-cord dysfunction presenting as asthma. *N Engl J Med*. 1983;308(26):1566–1570.
2. Kellman RM, Leopold DA. Paradoxical vocal cord motion: an important cause of stridor. *Laryngoscope*. 1982;92(1):58–60.
3. Barnes SD, Grob CS, Lachman BS, Marsh BR, Loughlin GM. Psychogenic upper airway obstruction presenting as refractory wheezing. *J Pediatr*. 1986;109(6):1067–1070.
4. Butani L, O'Connell EJ. Functional respiratory disorders. *Ann Allergy Asthma Immunol*. 1997;79(2):91–99; quiz 99–101.
5. Lacy TJ, McManis SE. Psychogenic stridor. *Gen Hosp Psychiatry*. 1994;16(3):213–223.
6. Wilson JJ, Wilson EM. Practical management: vocal cord dysfunction in athletes. *Clin J Sport Med*. 2006;16(4):357–360.
7. Balkissoon R, Kenn K. Asthma: vocal cord dysfunction (VCD) and other dysfunctional breathing disorders. *Semin Respir Crit Care Med*. 2015;33(6):595–605.

CHAPTER 4

Airway Fire

Why Are They Called "Laser-Resistant" Tubes?

Timothy D. Anderson

THE CASE

The patient was a 58-year-old male with multiple chronic medical problems (bedridden, rheumatoid arthritis, dialysis, diabetes, chronic obstructive pulmonary disease [COPD], etc) who had a tracheotomy placed due to long-term ventilation requirements due to respiratory failure. He was weaned from the ventilator, but the rehabilitation hospital was unable to cap the tracheotomy, and the patient was unable to speak or use a speaking valve. In addition, the patient had chronic aspiration and was G-tube dependent. Office laryngoscopy showed normal vocal fold motion, aspiration, and copious secretions below the vocal folds. Exam under anesthesia revealed a 99% dense, long tracheal stenosis. Trial of balloon dilation was unsuccessful. After prolonged discussion with the patient and his family, the primary goal of treatment was to regain the ability to communicate.

TREATMENT PLANNING

Due to the patient's rheumatoid arthritis and severe finger deformities, nonsurgical options were not ideal (Table 4–1). The patient was felt to be a poor candidate for tracheal resection due to his poor wound healing and multiple medical comorbidities, as well as the length of stenosis. Laryngectomy would be a reasonable option and would have the potential to rehabilitate both voice and swallowing, but the patient and family were against ablative surgery unless necessary. The decision was therefore made to proceed with a trial of endoscopic CO_2 laser debulking with the goal of re-establishing continuity of the trachea to allow for communication. The patient was aware that decanulation of the tracheotomy would not be possible with this procedure.

Table 4–1. Management Options

Nonsurgical	Surgical
Nonoral communication (writing, text-to-speech)	Endoscopic stenosis debulking
	Tracheal resection
Electrolarynx	Laryngectomy/trachea-esophageal prosthesis

THE PROCEDURE

The patient was brought to the operating room and intubated with a Xomed LaserShield II endotracheal tube through his tracheostomy stoma. A laryngoscope was inserted and used to expose the subglottis, and a rigid suction was passed through the eccentric stenosis and into the normal lower trachea. Both the suction and the normal cricoid cartilage were used as a guide, and the dense stenosis was gradually incised and removed by a combination of CO_2 laser and cold instruments. The endotracheal tube was frequently removed, and the direction and extent of surgery were frequently verified from both above and below the stenotic area.

FIRST ERROR OF JUDGMENT (SURGICAL)

During one of the endotracheal tube removals, the cuff was accidentally ruptured. A second laser-resistant tube was already in the room, and the tube was replaced. Unfortunately, when the cuff of the second tube was ruptured by scissors near the end of the case, a third laser-resistant tube was not immediately available. As the case was almost complete and cold instruments were being used, the decision was made to continue the case with the same tube despite the cuff rupture.

SECOND ERROR OF JUDGMENT (COMMUNICATION)

During the case, due to the patient's underlying lung disease and periods of apnea due to tube removal, the anesthesiologist gradually increased the inspired oxygen percentage to maintain oxygenation. After the second cuff rupture, with a nearly completely opened stenosis, ventilation became more difficult, and the inspired oxygen percentage was increased to nearly 100%. A 2-way failure of communication occurred, where the surgeon was unaware of the increased FiO_2, and the anesthesiologist was unaware of the fire risk.

THIRD ERROR OF JUDGMENT (KNOWLEDGE)

A final segment of granulation tissue was found, hanging down from just above the tracheotomy stoma. To minimize bleeding, the CO_2 laser was used to ablate it. The laser passed through the granulation and hit the deflated cuff in an oxygen-enhanced environment, causing an instant flash fire just below the stoma. As per protocol, the surgeon immediately yelled "fire," the scrub nurse poured saline into the laryngoscope, and the anesthesiologist removed the endotracheal tube. The fire was immediately extinguished but examination of the endotracheal tube (Figure 4–1) showed complete consumption of the cuff by fire and examination of the trachea showed superficial char and underlying erythema (Figure 4–2). The patient was re-intubated and weaned from anesthesia. He was observed overnight due to the risk of delayed edema and lung or airway damage. The fire was immediately disclosed to the patient's family, and to the patient once he was awake.

SURGICAL FIRES

Although surgical fires are uncommon (~1:500,000 surgeries), 23% of otolaryngologists report having had at least one surgical fire.[1] Surgical fires require an ignition source, fuel, and oxidizer. Possible ignition sources include electrocautery

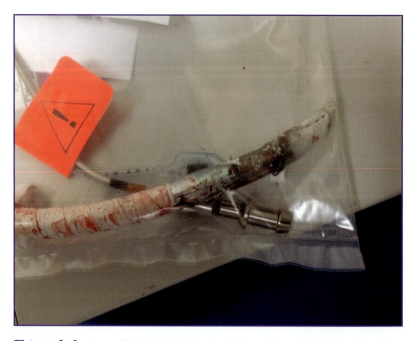

Figure 4–1. Laser Shield II endotracheal tube with cuff inflated with saline and close-up of cuff area after fire.

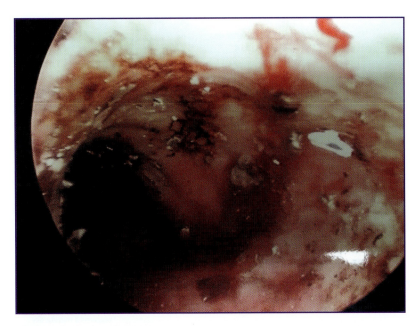

Figure 4–2. Superficial burns of trachea immediately below stoma.

(58% to 90%), endoscopic light cords (can heat to 670°F, up to 38% of fires), and CO_2 laser (3% to 13%, most common airway fire source).[2,3] The most common oxidizer is oxygen, and at high oxygen concentrations, even normally inert substances can become flammable. The fuel can be an endotracheal tube, red rubber catheter, paper drapes, or surgical sponge in the operative field.

WHAT I LEARNED FROM THIS CASE

Hospital Policy

Prior to this case, fire risk in the operating room was classified as low or high. High fire risk was any case in which a potential ignition source was used. This made virtually every otolaryngology case "high risk" but did not distinguish between cases such as this one with a truly high risk, and a case such as sinus surgery, where an endoscopic light cord was used, but the risk of significant fire was actually much lower. Because most otolaryngology cases were "high" fire risk, truly dangerous cases were not appropriately identified. This led to a change in hospital policy with a new "extreme" fire risk category added (Figure 4–3).

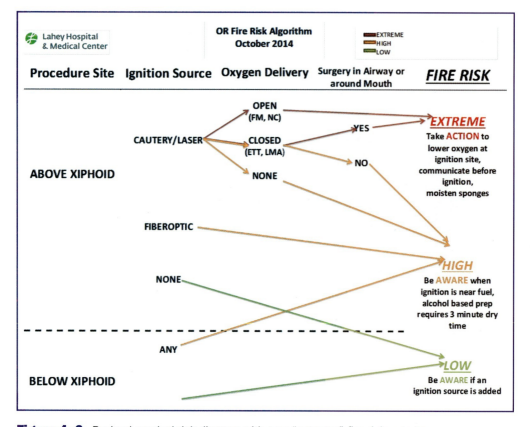

Figure 4–3. Revised surgical risk diagram with new "extreme" fire risk category.

Communication

As the operating surgeon, ultimate responsibility (and liability) for surgical fires rests with you. The surgeon is the one who best understands and controls the fire risk; it is therefore incumbent upon the surgeon to constantly communicate with the rest of the surgical team regarding fire risk, expectations for oxygen levels, and reduction of fuel in the surgical field. The surgical team, including the anesthesiologist, must in turn communicate regarding changing situations and patient factors.

Equipment

The endotracheal cuff of most laser-resistant tubes is made of flammable material and can be ignited by the CO_2 laser even when fully inflated with water.[4] Cases where the endotracheal tube is inserted through a tracheostomy stoma may expose more of the cuff and increase the risk of this type of fire. Unlike penetration of the tube lumen, there is no active oxygen flow through this portion of the tube, so distal tracheal injuries are less likely, but local tracheal burns can occur.

Training

Our hospital has an annual "surgical fire drill" that is required for all surgical staff. Causes and responses to surgical fires are reviewed at this meeting annually. The surgical team responded quickly and appropriately to the fire, quickly dousing the fire and preventing severe injury. Training with regular re-training is important to allow rapid and accurate team response to a rare event, such as a surgical fire.

CASE OUTCOME

The patient was observed overnight and had no airway complications. Re-examination of the trachea several days after the fire showed complete healing of the charred areas without further stenosis. He had an excellent result from the surgery and was not only able to use a speaking valve on his tracheotomy, but also had improvement in his swallow and resumed some oral intake. The patient and his family were grateful for the care they received despite the complication.

REFERENCES

1. Hempel S, Gibbons MM, Nguyen D, et al. Prevention of wrong site surgery, retained surgical items, and surgical fires: a systematic review. *VA Evidence-Based Synthesis Program Reports*, Department of Veterans Affairs: 2013.
2. Overbey DM, Townsend NT, Chapman BC, et al. Surgical energy-based device injuries and fatalities reported to the Food and Drug Administration. *J Am Coll Surg*. 2015;221(1):197–205.
3. Mehta SP, Bhananker SM, Posner KL, Domino KB. Operating room fires: a closed claims analysis. *Anesthesiology*. 2013;118(5): 1133–1139.
4. MAUDE Adverse Event Report: Medtronic Xomed Inc. Laser Shield II endotracheal tube BSK—cuff, tracheal tube, inflatable. http://www.accessdata.fda.gov/scripts/cdrh/cfdocs/cfmaude/detail.cfm?mdrfoi__id=1815162

SECTION 2

Risk Management

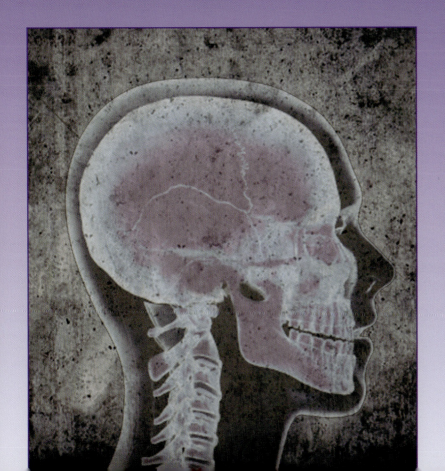

CHAPTER 5

The Uninsured Patient

Maintaining the Standard of Care

Wendy B. R. Stern

THE CASE

A 62-year-old male presented to my office for the first time with a chief complaint of nasal obstruction. In fact, it was so bad that "a balloon" kept popping out of the left side of his nose, and he had to keep pushing it back in! He worked as a self-employed landscaper and found this to be quite debilitating. His history was significant for prior sinus surgery and a total thyroidectomy for thyroid cancer. He was a nonsmoker, had no underlying medical conditions, and was not taking any medication other than thyroid hormone replacement. He was not allergic to any medications. On examination he had bilateral nasal polyps worse on the left side (Figure 5–1).

We discussed medical options and then had an in-depth discussion of the surgical management including the risks and benefits. In the end, he determined that his nasal breathing was critical to his ability to perform strenuous work and wished to further explore his surgical option. I ordered a

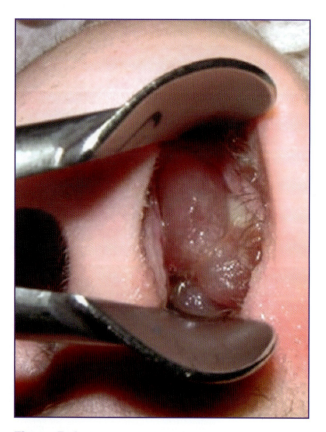

Figure 5–1. Left nasal polyps on anterior rhinoscopy.

preoperative sinus computed tomography (CT) and arranged a follow-up appointment. At the conclusion of the visit he mentioned that he did not have insurance. I advised him that both my office and the hospital would set up a fair payment plan. He returned shortly thereafter to review the sinus CT (Figure 5–2) and after a detailed discussion about the surgery chose a date for the procedure the following month.

He underwent bilateral endoscopic resection of nasal polyps, maxillary sinus antrostomies with removal of contents, and ethmoidectomy. The surgery was uneventful. Prior to the first postoperative appointment my office manager advised me that he had set up a payment plan. He was doing well with it, but it was going to take him a long time to complete his obligation.

So . . . in comes my patient. He is feeling great, so good he hopes not to have to come back again. We make a postoperative management plan and sometime during that discussion I am struck with a great idea. I have a yard and he is a landscaper. I ask him, "What do you think of the idea of coming by and doing yard work valued at what you owe me instead of this payment plan we've set up?" It sounded like a win/win situation to both of us. The last time I saw that patient for this episode of care, we were standing side by side in my yard doing the fall cleanup. He was still feeling great.

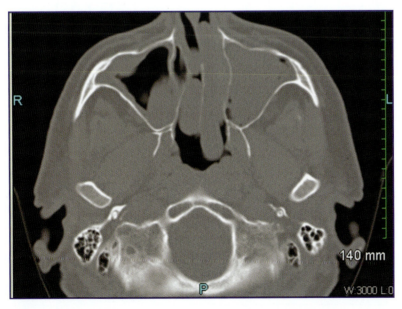

Figure 5–2. Axial sinus CT scan showing obstructive nasal polyps and sinus opacification.

THE CASE CONTINUES

Eighteen months later, this patient returns to my office with a new complaint. His right ear has been plugged for a couple of months in spite of being compliant with his irrigations and topical steroid nasal spray. He has a few ideas of his own as to the cause of his problem including occupational loud noise exposure. I examined him and noted a right serous otitis media (SOM). We discussed possible causes of unilateral SOM including eustachian tube dysfunction, recurrent polyps, and a nasopharyngeal mass. I performed fiberoptic nasopharyngoscopy and found his exam to be normal including well-healed sinus cavities. I did an audiogram (Figure 5–3) demonstrating a conductive hearing loss on the right and performed a myr-

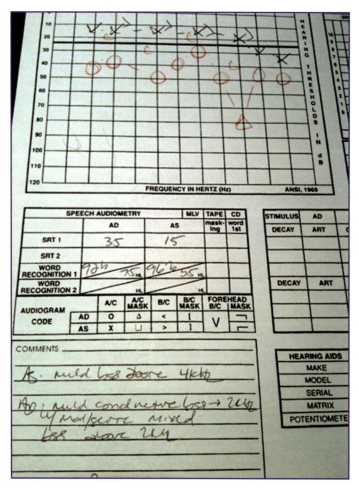

Figure 5–3. Audiogram with right conductive hearing loss.

ingotomy and aspiration of the right ear during this first visit with a follow-up appointment in 1 week.

And, by the way, I only charged him for an office visit. After all, he is a nice guy.

He did return the following week because things were a little worse. He was hearing better but now described a tingling and numbness around his right ear and face, and he was not feeling well. He had some more probable explanations. He was in the midst of dental work. He wondered if this could be Lyme disease or recurrent thyroid cancer, but his primary care physician had tested him and the lab work returned as normal.

GETTING SCARIER

Well, hopefully you (and I!) are getting a little bit scared by now. We discussed the differential diagnosis, and I advised him that he must get magnetic resonance imaging (MRI) to rule out skull base disease and set up an MRI with a 1-week follow-up appointment. He returned for the appointment but had not gone for the MRI. He didn't want to incur the expense and had realized that his symptoms could be from a Q-tip injury. Also, his dentist told him it could be of dental origin. On examination it was noted that he had a recurrent SOM on the right. I placed a tube this time and stressed the importance of the MRI and rescheduling the test and a follow-up appointment.

He didn't get the MRI or keep the next appointment and returned 1 month later when his symptoms worsened. It was noted that the tube was in place and functional, and again we discussed the importance of an MRI. The MRI (Figure 5–4) was finally obtained 2½ months after his initial presentation.

A large heterogeneous mass was noted to extend from the right sphenoid sinus into the posterior nasopharynx and into the pterygoid space with some bony erosion. On nasal endoscopy I could see a fleshy tumor arising from the right ethmoid complex. We discussed the findings. I recommended urgent biopsy and scheduled the surgery for a few days later.

Now, this is really scary. I find myself thinking back to the original surgery. Did I send gross or microscopic pathology? Did I miss the tumor? How well is my chart documented? The bottom line is, did I cut any corners trying to save on medical expense? I distract myself from my anxiety as I am performing the biopsy of this ugly tumor by telling the operating room team of the story of what a nice guy he is and how I operated

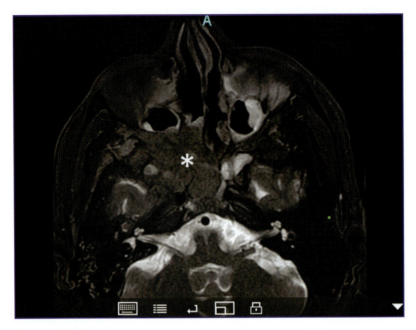

Figure 5–4. MRI of the head demonstrating right skull base mass.

on him before and how his workup got delayed because he didn't want to pay for the MRI. I then tell them the story about how he doesn't have insurance. As I am telling the story of how I bartered my services for his, the anesthesiologist looks up and says, *"That's illegal!"* Great! So what am I going to be sued for—misdiagnosis, the delay of diagnosis, or bartering?

CASE OUTCOME

It turns out that I did have microscopic pathology from the original surgery demonstrating normal polyp disease (Figure 5–5A). The mass turned out to be a large B-cell lymphoma (Figure 5–5B).

He had a total body positron emission tomography (PET) CT scan that revealed localized disease only. He was treated with rituximab, cyclophosphamide, doxorubicin, vincristine, and prednisone (R-CHOP), and intrathecal methotrexate. His posttreatment CT demonstrated a persistent mass in the right sphenoid sinus (Figure 5–6). He underwent right sphenoidotomy and removal of the mass that turned out to be a mucocele.

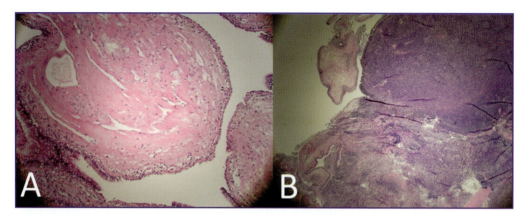

Figure 5–5. **A.** Pathology from the first sinus surgery demonstrating a benign inflammatory polyp. **B.** Pathology from the second endoscopic biopsy demonstrating large B-cell lymphoma.

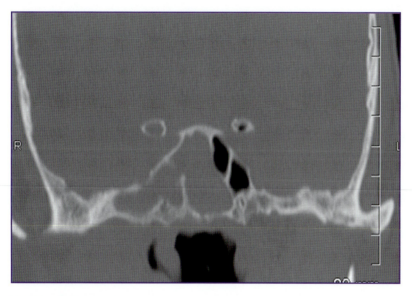

Figure 5–6. Posttreatment coronal CT scan of the sphenoid sinus demonstrating opacification of the right sphenoid sinus.

The remainder of his course was uneventful, and he is alive and well today. I haven't been sued for anything, but as I reflect, I wonder how I got into this scary situation. I consulted with experts who informed me that bartering is legal as long as you indicate on your tax returns the value of the services you received.

WHY WAS I IN THIS SITUATION?

There is tremendous pressure to reduce medical cost, not only to help the uninsured patient, but for all patients as our nation and Congress pursue efforts to consolidate medical care and reduce overall costs. Although the emphasis is to improve the quality of care, the focus on reduction of cost remains a central feature. We all understand that doing less is the fastest means to achieve this goal. Be wary! Always maintain the standard of care and consider existing guidelines and consensus statements when treating patients. Finally, utilize existing resources when helping the uninsured. Most hospital and health care organizations have social and financial services that can help your patient navigate the health care system.

ASK THE EXPERT: Anthony Abeln, JD

Can you barter for medical care? Can you not charge a patient for services? Does not charging change your legal liability?

There is no clear guidance on the scope of bartering for medical services. There are definitely some traps for the unwary, however. There are, for example, tax implications for some doctors—how would you go about declaring on your taxes the value received? There are federal laws that prevent the waiver of Medicare or Medicaid co-payments and deductibles or the acceptance of anything more or less valuable than the service provided. Any bartering should be valued and documented in accordance with the services or goods rendered.

That said, for the uninsured and those with private insurance, there are some doctors and clinics and even some companies that include medical and dental care among a larger barter system. It's important to check with your local medical society or licensing board for specifics in your state of licensure because state regulations can vary.

The key question, however, relative to specific care in this case is whether, in providing care for trade, this patient was treated the same way as any other patient who was billed in a traditional way for services. Imagine the question at a deposition—"If this patient had paid you or held adequate health insurance, would you, Doctor, have indicated that he needed any other tests? Would you have recommended any other procedures? Would you have performed tests more rapidly? Offered any other office-based treatments?" The essence of the case is whether you provided the standard of care despite the method, or lack thereof, of payment.

Even if the patient does not pay you, but you maintain a physician-patient relationship, in most cases, that patient is still *your* patient, and you have all of the responsibilities that you would for any other patient regardless of outstanding debts.

CHAPTER 6

Facial Plastic Surgery

The Case Without End

Jeffrey H. Spiegel

When the editors of this book asked me to contribute a chapter in which I needed to describe the events of a "scary" case in the practice of facial plastic surgery, I initially drew a blank. Short of Michael Jackson's nose and a few Hollywood starlets, what could be frightening about facial plastic surgery? A missed tee time? (Or missed "tea time" for our colleagues in the United Kingdom). Having to answer a phone call on the weekend?

However, upon further reflection I realized that much of the daily work of a facial plastic surgeon would be considered scary to many, and with a shudder was able to dredge from the dark recesses of my mind the following dark tale. I suggest reading this with the lights fully on, and not late at night.

I present to you:

THE CASE WITHOUT END

It was a dark and stormy night. Well, probably anyway. Some of those details are lost, and it's unlikely I was seeing patients at night. Nonetheless, at some point a 57-year-old woman came to see me with complaints regarding looking older.

She was a pack-a-day smoker, and she looked like it. She had the deep facial rhytids, heavy neck banding, and windburned facial skin of a longshoreman with a voice to match.

During our discussion, I learned that she had recently ended a long and tumultuous relationship and was looking to make a "fresh start." This sounded reasonable; many people look to get plastic surgery around significant life events: a big birthday, a divorce, prior to a personal or professional transition. The termination of a bad relationship seemed a reasonable time to take stock of one's life, determine new goals, and take the first steps toward self-actualization.

There was a lot of work to do. She needed to stop smoking, and this was but the most obvious way her life choices were self-defeating. We discussed the aging process. We discussed healthy habits. We discussed my recommendations (which were extensive, well considered, and truly insightful but for the sake of brevity let's just say that we decided she would have a facelift). Then we reviewed the limitations of plastic surgery, and we discussed the risks.

In addition to having a comprehensive consent form that specifically lists any potential risk of surgery I can think of, I always go over risks in direct conversation at least three times before surgery (at the consultation, at a preoperative visit, and on the morning of surgery). Then, I go over any remaining risks after surgery as well (such as prolonged healing, late-forming hematoma, etc).

Yes, she was a smoker, but she agreed that her desire for a fresh start and to have a rhytidectomy were strong motivation for smoking cessation. There are various studies that suggest the proper time frame for smoking cessation prior to surgery, and we used a safe margin. I stressed to her that smoking would limit the extent of correction she could expect, could affect her healing, and may increase her hematoma risk.

So, having properly prepared my patient, eaten a nutritious breakfast (me, not the patient), and scrubbed my hands, I did a facelift.

A hematoma formed.

No. No hematoma. I don't use drains either as they don't seem to correlate with a reduced incidence of hematoma. The key with hematoma prevention is to control blood pressure.[1]

The skin flaps necrosed.

No. Not that either. I was ready for that. She was a smoker so I adjusted the skin flap depth and length accordingly. We had thoroughly discussed that possibility, and while skin flap necrosis is disappointing and frustrating, it is not especially scary for the experienced surgeon or prepared patient.

Actually, everything went fine. She went home after surgery and came back to the office the next day. The flaps were flat, pink, and healthy looking. I changed her dressing and advised her about the next few days.

On postoperative day 7 she returned, and I removed her sutures and staples. I counseled her about patience, not overdoing it with her activity, and the expected results.

THE NEVER ENDING BEGINS

A few weeks later she returned, dissatisfied. "There has been no change," I was told along with, "what a waste of money." The most revealing, and honest, comment was actually the next one she offered: "Nothing is better."

I've seen this before. I often counsel patients that the most difficult part of facial plastic surgery is recognizing that they look better.

A Flashback

Many people know that I have an interest in facial feminization surgery and have taken care of thousands of transgender women with these procedures.[2–4] More than a decade before the facelift patient of whom I write came into my office, I consulted on a 24-year-old transgender woman from Europe who looked very masculine and was interested in full facial feminization surgery. She received full facial feminization surgery and looked great. She agreed.

As you may have anticipated, she returned stating she was, upon further reflection, displeased with her results. I objectively evaluated the outcome and felt she was doing well. She persisted in her complaints. Eager to please, I offered to adjust all aspects of her surgery in order to make her happy. This, I did, and she looked even better than before (and remember, she already looked great). She was now happy . . . until she wasn't. She wanted another complete revision.

I wanted her to be happy and would have done this. However, there was nothing left to do. Everything was right and at this point further surgery would be doing harm. I explained to her this limitation and apologized that I was unable to offer her more but expressed my sincere belief that she had achieved and surpassed her initial goals.

Then began endless e-mails, phone calls, and messages telling me how awful I was. That would have been a nice ending to this story. But it was not to be; the next part was that she created a webpage with a URL that can roughly be described as www.I-hate-DrSpiegel.com. As she was a computer professional, and I am not, her webpage soon had a greater Internet presence and more visitors than did my own webpage, innocently (and similarly) named http://www.DrSpiegel.com.

On this new webpage (http://www.I-hate-DrSpiegel.com) she described her experience with me and posted numerous before and after photographs of her surgeries in order to demonstrate to others her bad outcomes. Many people went to her site and reviewed the information. As a result my phone started ringing off the hook and dozens of new patients started booking surgery with me. It seems that even if she didn't see the benefits of surgery on her own face, others could appreciate the changes and wanted to look as "bad" as she did.

Once the dissatisfied patient learned of how her website was backfiring, she took it down. But the boost to my practice persisted. As an epilogue, about a year later she apologized for her actions and said she was happy. She related that her initial unhappiness was because after surgery she went back to her regular lonely life with a job she didn't like. And, what was it that enabled her to finally recognize that she looked good? She had a new boyfriend.

Back to the Scary Case, and Some People (Me) Never Learn

My facelift patient was unhappy and "nothing was improved." Objectively, she looked much better. Her jawline was more defined, her sagging neck skin was elevated, and her overall appearance was younger, healthier, and brighter . . . except for the perpetual frown.

So, what did I do? I spoke with her about expectations. I showed her before and after photos of her face from multiple angles. I reasoned with her. We re-evaluated after a few more weeks. Things were settling nicely. She had thin and fading scars. She had significant improvement. I would have been very confident showing her result to my peers or to prospective patients. So she changed tactics. Now came the threats. The negative reviews online followed along with a never-ending barrage of phone calls, complaints, e-mails, and messages that distracted and demoralized me and my staff in addition to consuming a tremendous amount of time. Somehow this situation had to stop.

I offered to do the facelift again.

In 1979 the R&B group Shalamar had a hit with the song "Second Time Around." You may remember the lyrics that included this verse:

> The second time around
> Ooh, the second time is so much better, baby
> The second time around
> Add I'll make it better than the first time

With that song in my head I redid the facelift. And it was better. As surgeons we're all taught some version of the old Italian aphorism that "Better Is the Enemy of Good." In this case, better was just better than good. The first time things came out well, and the second time they looked even better. The patient wasn't right that she needed a revision, but surely she would now be happy.

But she wasn't. I was heartbroken but with a sense of déjà vu. She complained at each visit. She came once with her sister who agreed that the results were great but said, "Oh, my sister is never satisfied with anything." Why didn't anyone tell me that beforehand?

At this point, the patient demanded a refund. She had paid for a facelift and gotten a good one, plus a second one on the house. She had received hours upon hours of high-quality care from my office. I said no.

Fortunately for me, she wasn't a computer programmer so she didn't have the wherewithal to create a disparaging website. She also wasn't of the right age to be familiar with how to criticize me in another online forum.

So, she decided to picket my office.

The patient informed us that if she didn't receive a refund, in full, she would begin picketing the front door of my medical practice (which is on the street level at a busy intersection) in order to prevent other people from coming to see me.

Now, she did hang around the front of the office for a while, but the weather in the Boston area can be unpleasant and she didn't last long. As it turns out there was not much picketing, and I later learned that during the period in which these events were unfolding she had not yet found a new boyfriend (as amazing as that seems for such a beautiful human being) and had other stressors in her life. Dr. Sigmund Sattenspiel, a facial plastic surgeon in New Jersey, once told me that in his experience, patients are never satisfied with their plastic surgery until they get, er, until they have a romantic encounter after healing. That may be right, but I'm not quite certain how to use that information to help my patients recognize their excellent outcomes. In any case, the patient had somewhat revealed the secret truth, for when she complained that "nothing is better" after surgery, she wasn't speaking about her appearance.

FADING AWAY

Eventually, the patient just lost interest in me, or realized she looked good and had nothing left to say. To paraphrase another old aphorism, a bad ending is better than badness without end.

There are many reasons why patients are dissatisfied with their plastic surgery. Sometimes the surgeon just didn't deliver the intended outcome (of course, not in my cases).

Other times the patients have unrealistic expectations, or a form of body dysmorphic disorder, but these can usually be identified in advance by an experienced physician.

Perhaps Ricky Nelson had the answer in his 1972 song, "Garden Party," when he sang:

> But it's all right now, I've learned my lesson well
> You see, you can't please everyone, so you've got to please yourself

We do want to please everyone, but you can only do your best. I've learned to inquire about my patients' "psycho-social-sexual history" in greater detail than I may want to know, and take solace in knowing that I truly want excellent outcomes for my patients. In fact, I tell each of my patients that just before surgery and I think it helps. I say:

"I want nothing more than to make you happy today. I'm going to do everything I know how to do in order to make certain that the surgery goes well and you come out with a safe, healthy, and beautiful result."

I'm not sure it will prevent one of these scary cases from happening again, but it can help two important people: the patient and the physician.

REFERENCES

1. Kleinberger AJ, Spiegel JH. What is the best method for minimizing the risk of hematoma formation after rhytidectomy? *Laryngoscope*. 2015 Mar;125(3):534–536. doi: 10.1002/lary.24685. Epub 2014 Apr 2
2. Spiegel JH. Facial determinants of female gender and feminizing forehead cranioplasty. *Laryngoscope*. 2011 Feb;121(2):250–261. doi: 10.1002/lary.21187. Epub 2010 Nov 30.
3. Ainsworth TA, Spiegel JH. Quality of life of individuals with and without facial feminization surgery or gender reassignment surgery. *Qual Life Res*. 2010 Sep;19(7):1019–1024. doi: 10.1007/s11136-010-9668-7.
4. Spiegel JH. Challenges in care of the transgender patient seeking facial feminization surgery. *Facial Plast Surg Clin North Am*. 2008 May;16(2):233–238, viii. doi: 10.1016/j.fsc.2007.11.011.

CHAPTER 7

Malingering

An Unusual Stapedectomy Outcome

Terry J. Garfinkle

THE CASE

A 33-year-old female G2P2 presented with a 2-year history of hearing loss and mild pulsatile tinnitus in the right ear. She had a documented conductive hearing loss on audiogram performed 1 year earlier. She denied a history of head trauma, previous otologic surgery, or vertigo. There was a positive family history of hearing loss in her father which had never been evaluated. The physical examination was unremarkable with the exception of tuning fork testing showing Weber lateralizing to the right ear and bone conduction greater than air conduction in the right ear. Audiologic evaluation confirmed a mixed hearing loss in the right ear with a 35 to 40 dB conductive component (Figure 7–1). Speech reception threshold (SRT) was 55 dB in the right ear and 20 dB in the left ear. Speech recognition scores were 100% bilaterally. The patient was thought to have a diagnosis of otosclerosis in the right ear.

The patient was presented with the therapeutic options of amplification versus surgical exploration with possible stapedectomy or ossiculoplasty based on the intraoperative findings. The potential risks and benefits of the procedure were fully explained and documented in the medical record. The patient underwent right middle ear exploration under local anesthesia with monitored intravenous sedation. The diagnosis of otosclerosis was confirmed, and a stapedectomy procedure was initiated. The stapes suprastructure was removed and the oval window opened, at which point the patient became restless

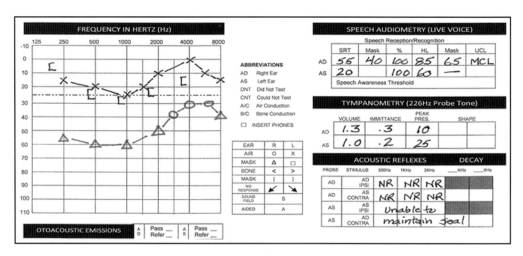

Figure 7–1. Preoperative audiogram showing unilateral conductive hearing loss consistent with otosclerosis.

and talkative but not complaining of pain or vertigo. Sedation was gently increased by the anesthesiologist but this resulted in increasing restlessness and agitation. The procedure could not be completed safely with this level of agitation so the oval window was plugged with previously harvested fat (from the earlobe) and the case was converted to general anesthesia. The patient was repositioned, re-prepped, and re-draped before resuming the procedure. The stapedectomy was then completed using a Shucknecht wire-piston, and fat was used to seal the oval window around the prosthesis.

FULL DISCLOSURE

The intraoperative events were shared with the patient that evening when she was alert. As might be anticipated, the patient had significant and persistent postoperative vertigo. She was discharged to home after 2 days and was seen in the office numerous times as well as followed regularly by phone over the ensuing 3 weeks. She had very little subjective improvement and Weber testing consistently lateralized to the surgical ear. The possibility of intraoperative labyrinthine injury was considered as a cause of her persisting vertigo, as was a persisting perilymphatic leak or a prosthesis of excessive length. The latter two being correctable, a recommendation for re-exploration was made given her failure to improve.

REVISION SURGERY

The patient returned to the operating room for re-exploration under general anesthesia. There was no perilymphatic fistula identified, but the prosthesis was felt to be too long. The 4.25 × 0.6 mm prosthesis was replaced with one measuring 4.0 × 0.6 mm. The patient had subjective improvement within several days and was seen several times within the first 2 weeks post-op.

TROUBLE BEGINS

The patient missed several consecutive appointments. We reached out to the patient to encourage follow-up. She returned 6 weeks after her second procedure with symptoms of mild residual vertigo and subjectively poor hearing in the right ear. Weber testing now lateralized to the contralateral ear! Audiogram suggested a severe to profound sensorineural hearing loss (SNHL) in the right ear with SRT of 70 dB!

A long conversation was held with the patient outlining the possible causes of this adverse outcome including the open vestibule during intraoperative intubation, re-opening of the vestibule during revision surgery and other unexplained causes. Sincerest apologies were expressed for the poor result. The patient seemed to accept the poor result and was surprisingly unconcerned. Vestibular therapy was arranged to help her with her residual symptoms and recommendations were made for a 6-month follow-up visit.

One month later we received a request from the patient for copies of her medical record. This request can often signal a second opinion, an unhappy patient, or initiation of a malpractice claim.

CASE OUTCOME

A week or so later, I received a call from a colleague at a nearby institution stating that the patient had been evaluated there and that there were some inconsistencies in her audiometric testing. Weber still lateralized to the contralateral ear and initial pure-tone thresholds were 75 to 95 dB, but speech reception thresholds had some inconsistencies on that day. Click-evoked auditory brainstem response (ABR) was performed revealing threshold of *35 dB in the right ear*! Repeat *pure-tone average was 17 dB in the right ear with complete closure of the air-bone gap*! When confronted with these good postoperative results by my cross-town colleague, both the patient and her mother displayed visible disappointment!?! I thanked my colleague profusely for her professionalism and assistance in uncovering the apparent deception.

As would be expected, the patient did not keep her appointments for vestibular therapy nor did she return to either office for follow-up.

THIS CASE WAS SCARY BECAUSE

This case was scary on several levels. First, the idiosyncratic response to increased sedation was unpredictable and quite concerning for completing a safe stapedectomy. Second, the conversion to general anesthesia after the vestibule was opened carries high risk for adverse outcome. Third, the patient experienced severe iatrogenic vertigo for an extended period of time after her procedure. Fourth, the patient required replacement of her prosthesis shortly after the original procedure, necessitating the re-opening of the vestibule, adding additional risk to both balance and hearing. Fifth, the patient appears to have had an adverse outcome from both a vestibular and acoustic perspective. This sets the stage for potential litigation. Finally, the patient appears to have been seeking secondary gain despite having a near-perfect outcome from her surgery.

WHAT I LEARNED FROM THIS CASE

In general, patients are truly appreciative of the efforts and sincere caring of their health care team. Most, however, does not mean *all*!

Appreciate your colleagues and maintain healthy and respectful relationships with them, as you will often see one another's clinical failures. Remain objective when evaluating a patient for a second opinion, and avoid the temptation to reflexively criticize your colleagues when they have an adverse outcome. You will have them as well!

Ask the Expert: Anthony Abeln, JD

How do you protect yourself from patients seeking secondary gains from malpractice claims? What if a patient is falsifying symptoms for personal gain?

One important question that comes up in many malpractice cases is how a follow-up treating physician has criticized the care that was provided at another institution. Two questions that such treaters need to ask themselves before they commit to such an assessment is, first, whether or not they have all of the information that they need in order to make an assessment as to whether or not a colleague may have made an error and, second, why the criticism is being made. Think of yourself in the position of an expert on the stand at a trial; do you have enough information to make a determination at the time that you criticize a fellow doctor for the care he or she has provided? Furthermore, to the extent that you do make such a criticism, what is your motivation? Of course, if you have an opinion based on your training, experience, and all of the information you need, and want to tell the patient that there was a problem in his or her prior care, you should do so; recognize, however, the seriousness of the allegation and how tightly a family may grab on to that going forward.

Furthermore, the words physicians use both in writing and in communicating to a patient are extremely important. Of course, patients who are getting second opinions (and their families) are understandably scared and concerned. An offhand remark, like "had this been caught earlier, something may have been done" can be interpreted as "this should have been caught earlier and it would have changed the outcome." Words matter!

If you feel as though your work is being used to support a claim against another provider, you can also consider two things. One, if the patient was not involved in a lawsuit (or if you did not suspect that), what would you do? Follow your normal course! Also, remember to document as much as you can of the encounter.

SUGGESTED READINGS

Han WW, Incesulu A, McKenna MJ, Rauch SD, Nadol JB, Jr, Glynn RJ. Revision stapedectomy: intraoperative findings, results, and review of the literature, *Laryngoscope.* 1997 Sep;107(9):1185–1192.

van Drie JC, van der Baan S, Bronkhorst AW, Feenstra L. Causes and results of reoperations following stapedectomy [Article in Dutch]. *Ned Tijdschr Geneeskd.* 1989 Aug 5;133(31):1546–1550.

Wegner I, Bittermann AJ, Zinsmeester MM, van der Heijden GJ, Grolman W. Local versus general anesthesia in stapes surgery for otosclerosis: a systematic review of the evidence. *Otolaryngol Head Neck Surg.* 2013 Sep;149(3):360–365. doi: 1177/0194599813493393. Epub 2013 Jun 13.

CHAPTER 8

Four Things to Keep in Mind to Make Those Scary Cases a Little Less Formidable

Anthony E. Abeln

Not surprisingly, there is no silver bullet that can prevent scary cases from occurring, and no magic charm to protect against lawsuits (whether frivolous or substantive) in your practice. What you can do is take a step back and review your practice and identify your strengths and weaknesses as a provider. That said, there are some general themes in practice that you can control that may help you sidestep some scary cases—and most of them are merely common sense:

1. Document, document, document, and when you're finished documenting, document more. There are rarely cases where too much documentation causes issues relative to a procedure that you have performed or chosen not to perform; more often than not, issues arise when there is a lack of documentation—for example, the scope of informed consent, documentation of a patient's history, who was present for the surgery, and so on.
2. Communicate, communicate, communicate: In so many depositions and trials, attorneys hear stories told by patients that the doctor wasn't available to communicate, to call him or her, that the doctor wouldn't come and see us in a hospital, that the doctor sent a resident instead of coming himself or herself to check on the patient. If the family feels as though you as the patient's physician were being attentive, over time, they are certainly more likely to favorably view the care that you provided.

    Remember that these vulnerable family members and friends, faced with an unexpected injury to a loved one, understandably take these initial conversations very seriously. How the physician presents himself or herself and the words that the physician uses during these delicate conversations matter.

    In recent depositions of physicians, I've seen plaintiffs angry that the physician "couldn't wait to get out of the room." Plaintiffs describe physicians who describe what happened in the operating room as a "plane crash." Wives describe how primary care providers seemed uninterested in the admission of their husbands. Patients describe how physicians are callous about their recovery.

    Spending a few more minutes, answering as many questions as you can, and showing extra patience to a family member may not inoculate you from a lawsuit,

but it certainly will help in allaying concerns that a patient might have.
3. Did I mention document?
4. Engage with your colleagues about scary cases. Most scary cases are even scarier when they are looked at in a vacuum. A chronic problem among professionals—and attorneys are among the worst offenders—is that they don't want to discuss scary cases, particularly ones where they might face the judgment of their peers. But at the same time, medical professionals can come to second guess their own practice. Medical peer review processes make clear in some jurisdictions, there is a camaraderie in knowing that what you have gone though (or are going through) isn't something that you are facing alone. Also, there are a good number of mental health professionals who focus on helping professionals manage the stress associated with litigation that arises out of scary cases.

I would be remiss, moreover, if I did not try to exorcise any potential scary cases myself with the following . . .

Nothing in the above statements or in any of the above commentary should be deemed to be the provision of legal advice or counsel, or to in any way imply a standard of care related to any federal, state, or local matter. Any discussion of legal matters should be taken as points of further discussion and not to be any way relied upon as legal counsel. Please seek legal advice in your own jurisdiction relative to any and all of the issues that have arisen out of any of the "Scary Cases" herein. In point of fact, it's probably best to completely ignore anything written by Abeln . . .

CHAPTER 9

Malpractice Defense From the Expert Witness Perspective

R. William Mason

My career as an expert witness defending physicians started when I myself was sued. While seeing patients one afternoon, a gentleman approached me, and without introduction, handed me an envelope, stating, "I'm sorry to deliver this, Doc." I called in the next patient, and decided, with much difficulty and self-restraint, to open it at the end of the day.

As expected, it was a subpoena for my medical records. The patient was an elderly woman who suffered a facial nerve injury during mastoid surgery. I knew the case—had been thinking about it off and on for some time. What could I have done differently? Had the post-op complication been handled to the best of my ability? Had I been there for the patient, and her extended family? All of these questions again ran through my mind as I looked down at the subpoena.

The first thing I learned, you are never prepared for the emotional toll that a subpoena brings with it. We are all trained to care for our patients in a competent and skilled manner. Yet here was a document accusing me of negligence, in failing in my responsibilities to my patient. The next day, I called my malpractice carrier. They were sympathetic. These calls are an everyday occurrence to them—if not to me.

Learning point number two—this is just business, about money and compensation.

"Doctor, it's not personal." You will hear that over and over. Yet it was most personal, an affront to my skill and caring as a doctor. No, it is personal.

The next step was to closely review the chart. A word of advice. DO NOT ALTER YOUR CHART. It is no longer yours, but a legal document. I have reviewed cases that were clearly defensible but were settled due to someone changing the chart. One well-meaning medical secretary, unknown to her boss, meticulously altered the record, using three different pens! Plaintiff's attorney knew we couldn't go to court and pushed for settlement in the amount of the maximum malpractice coverage—one million dollars. The case: sensorineural hearing loss following otitis externa. Most likely pre-existing, and clearly unrelated to the treatment of an otitis externa. And yet it eventually settled. So do not alter the chart. It is no longer yours but is now a legal document.

Next, a meeting with the attorney. I couldn't schedule the meeting soon enough. Here was my defender—who would let them know, beyond a shadow of a doubt, that I had done no wrong. Well, not exactly. We went over the facts in the case in great detail. Most important, he informed me that this case would go on for years, sometimes as long as 5 years.

First would come discovery, where all documents would be forwarded to plaintiff's attorney. Next would be a presentation by plaintiff's attorney to a tribunal, required in the State of Massachusetts to prove that this was a valid case. A brief hope, quickly dashed, when I was told that the bar was quite low—if they had a plaintiff's expert, that was enough to move forward with the case. The case would not be judged on its merits at this juncture. Next would come depositions. Probably a good year away. His advice: don't discuss the case with anyone, and don't give it any more thought until we come to the deposition. Good advice. Hard to accomplish.

You will go over this case many times in the next year—while driving your car, walking your dog, laying in bed at night. "Will I lose my house? My reputation?" It will occupy your thoughts. Yet, in retrospect, this was sound advice. There is absolutely nothing you can do at this stage. If you can, file it away until further notice. A Zen-like discipline. Worth developing, for many reasons, not all of them related to litigation.

True to form, the deposition came up 14 months later. This was what I had been waiting for. A chance to defend myself. After hearing my side, they would probably drop the case for lack of merit. *Wrong.* This is simply information gathering. You are welcomed into a well-appointed conference room, given a cup of coffee, greeted by a pleasant man who assures you that this is nothing personal. Again.

Resist the temptation to go into detail. The best deposition I have ever reviewed as a defense expert was quite brief. The doc made no effort to justify his actions or decisions, and limited his answers to "Yes, no, I don't know, I can't recall." Perfect! This is a fishing expedition. The more you talk, the greater the chance of some small detail showing up on your cross-examination in court. "Doctor, didn't you day this during your deposition? Well, wouldn't that indicate . . . " So resist all attempts to justify your actions. "Yes. No. I don't recall."

And don't *ever* lose your temper. Simply request a bathroom break and have a word with your lawyer. A general rule of the universe: you never win an argument with a lawyer. Maybe unless you are married to one. But maybe not even then.

Well, the deposition has come and gone. You will be asked to review the deposition. This is simply to identify misspellings, and not to elaborate upon your answers. Time to put the case out of your mind—again. If you can, this is the best advice I can give. Keep in mind, *the vast majority of malpractice cases that go to trial are won by the defendant.*

Fast-forward a few years. Now you are getting ready for trial. In my own case, I couldn't put it out of my mind, no matter how hard I tried. So I started doing my own research. I even met with the medical illustrator to help design the "chalks," the diagrams that are used at trial. My reasoning was that I would be using them to describe the relevant anatomy, and therefore wanted some say in the design of the illustrations. My attorney was absolutely supportive of these efforts. So another word of advice: at this juncture, become involved in your defense. You are the best expert the jury will hear from.

In my own case, while enduring a grueling cross-examination from plaintiff's attorney, I asked if I could get out of the witness box to illustrate a point with a chalk. Plaintiff's attorney immediately jumped up. "I object. He is the defendant, not the expert." The judge looked down his glasses at him, as one would examine a small bug, and overruled. Fact. The judge, the jury, and any observers in the courtroom are on your side. People will believe a doctor before they will believe a lawyer. Or even the plaintiff's expert. Or maybe even your expert. But they do want to hear from you. And believe you.

Once I got out of the witness box, I became a teacher, and not a defendant. Very powerful. As much as you have been dreading this day, this is your time to shine. To explain how complex medicine can be, how we make decisions, how we do surgery. The jury will be sitting on the edge of their seats. This is what they want to hear—an intimate view into the secret world of medicine. And you are their guide.

After the verdict, in our favor, my attorney took me aside. Would you consider being an expert witness? Shocked, I asked what my qualifications would be. That I had been sued? His answer was very revealing. He liked that

- I was closely involved in the preparation of the case.
- I came across to the jury as caring and professional.
- I was able to explain complex concepts and details in a manner that a layman could understand.
- And probably most important: "You didn't give it up on cross."

A word about that last point. When you are on the stand, either as an expert witness or a defendant, on direct exam you will look like a professor. But on cross-examination, every effort will be made to make you angry, question your testimony, look for inconsistencies, and lead you into some form of trap. "Well doctor, if A is true, and you've agreed to B, then doesn't that lead to C?" The calm answer: "No, I wouldn't agree to that." During cross-examination, you won't score many points. But if plaintiff's attorney pitches you one low and slow—by all means, hit it out of the park. For those of you who are considering becoming an expert witness, some advice. A good expert witness has three different hats that he or she wears.

One: A detective. Read the chart with attention to *every* detail. We once won a case based on one line in a nurse's note: "Patient says he has had difficulty swallowing for years."

Two: A writer. You will be asked to write a chronology and summary. This is your chance to stand up for the defendant. Make it convincing. Explain in common language why these actions and outcomes did not indicate negligence. Your message: "Don't settle this one!"

Three: An actor. On the stand, you are not a doctor. You're an actor playing a doctor. You carry no authority based on your title, just the ability to explain the facts in a caring and clear manner. And then hold up on cross. As a doctor, no one treats us this way. On cross, you will tested. Just keep smiling. And don't engage.

In closing, I am often asked: do you testify against doctors? I do, and for several reasons. First, you may be the first one to review a claim against a fellow physician. This is an opportunity to educate plaintiff's attorney as to the strength, if any, of his or her claim of negligence. I have found that there are two types of plaintiff's attorney.

The first, upon hearing a marginally supportive review, and after hearing that a strong defense argument would be presented, asks, "But doc, would you be comfortable saying . . . " The answer should be an emphatic "no." If I was comfortable with that statement, I would have said it.

The second thanks you for your review, and after hearing defense objections to his claim of negligence, decides not to go forward with the case. In this instance, you have performed a valuable service to the attorney, saving him or her time and money on a case that he or she would most likely lose. And most important, you have performed a service to your fellow physician.

Having said that, although 98% of my expert witness work is for defense counsel, I do believe we have an obligation to educate a jury in cases where negligence may be a factor. To fail in this responsibility is not a service to our profession.

In closing, I would say that serving as an expert witness has provided much satisfaction throughout my career, with an added benefit of continuing my education into the art and science of medicine. If after giving it some thought, you would consider serving as an expert witness, I would emphatically say: do it! After all, my sole qualification was that I had been sued.

SECTION 3

Medical Ethics

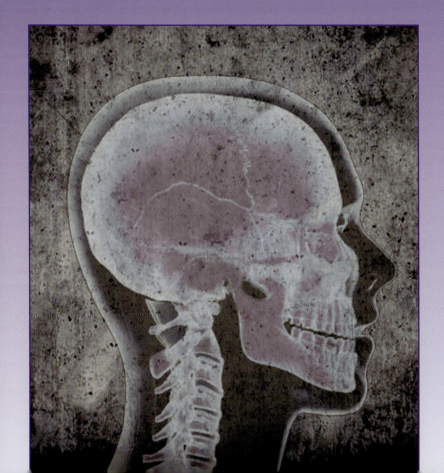

CHAPTER 10

Decision-Making Capacity

You Don't Want to Have Surgery, But You Have to Have Surgery

Kevin S. Emerick

THE CASE

A 65-year-old man was admitted for a right temple region lesion. He was found on the street by the Healthcare for Homeless team and brought into the hospital for further evaluation and care. He did not resist coming to the hospital but was not particularly concerned about the lesion. He reported it was relatively new and was not causing him any trouble. Upon review of his medical record, this was not a new lesion. Two years prior to this admission he was seen at another hospital in the city. At that time he had been admitted under similar circumstances by another team of health care providers for homeless patients. The lesion at that time by report was smaller than its current size but still several centimeters in diameter. He was admitted to the hospital to help facilitate management of the lesion, and a biopsy revealed cutaneous squamous cell carcinoma. Surgical excision was recommended; however, he refused treatment.

Based on reports from the Healthcare for Homeless team and the outside hospital notes, the patient had a long psychiatric history including bipolar disorder with delusions. He was well known to many of the homeless shelters and Healthcare for Homeless providers in the area. However, he had not been involved in any formal treatment programs and primarily lived on the street. His previous admission notes suggested he was very resistant to any traditional medical therapies including treatment for his bipolar disorder. Little else was known about him, and he provided no additional information about his personal or medical history.

At the time of his admission to the outside hospital, he clearly stated his desire not to have treatment. He was planning to seek alternative treatment strategies. He was convinced that there was a laser treatment option available that was being withheld from him. During that admission he was seen by the psychiatry team and deemed competent to make decisions. With this assessment made, he chose to leave the hospital without any treatment and never followed up. He did not have any care in the intervening 2 years and was intermittently in and out of various homeless shelters. On the evening of admission he was found by one of the Healthcare for Homeless teams on the street. They noted a large fungating lesion with maggots in the wound. Given the overall picture and inability to care for himself, he was brought to the hospital for further management.

At the time of the admission he had a 15-cm lesion involving the right temple region. Computed tomography (CT) imaging was performed and demonstrated a deeply infiltrative lesion. It extended well beyond the subcutaneous fat to involve the zygoma and the parotid fascia. Clinically the tumor was ulcerative in nature with rounded borders. The frontal branch of his facial nerve was clinically involved causing complete paralysis of the ipsilateral forehead. There was also palpable adenopathy in the parotid region and CT imaging suggested metastatic nodes in the parotid gland. A multidisciplinary Head and Neck Oncology team was convened to discuss all available treatment options. The team recommended the common treatment for this type of metastatic tumor, namely, surgical resection and adjuvant radiation.

Similar to his previous admission at the outside hospital, the patient refused surgery. He insisted on finding a laser treatment, topical treatment, or other "potion" to cure the cancer. He was very clear in his words about not wanting surgery. Unlike his previous admission, the psychiatry team on this occasion did not feel that he was competent to make decisions and a court-appointed guardian was put into place. Through all of this, the patient was well cared for by the nursing staff, many of whom were very fond of the patient.

At this point, important decisions had to be made to help direct care. The patient did not want surgery and the nurses on the floor felt it was wrong to proceed with surgery. The nurses felt strongly that surgery was wrong because he stated so clearly how he did not want a surgical intervention. The oncology team weighed the natural history of the lesion; further progression locally leading to increased wound issues, complete facial nerve paralysis, and eventual death from uncontrolled local and regional progression versus the patient's desire to avoid conventional treatments. The psychiatry team felt the patient was not competent to make decisions and that standard of care should not be withheld from the patient. Last, the court-appointed guardian also felt that standard of care should be provided to the patient, and it was wrong to allow this patient to die of uncontrolled disease when he could not understand the consequences of his decision not to undergo treatment. A last challenge to this decision came when the local police department asked to have the patient fingerprinted. The social security number provided by the patient belonged to a woman four states away. We did not know who this patient was.

THIS CASE WAS SCARY BECAUSE

This case was scary because of the multiple divergent opinions on how best to manage this case. There was a strong desire from all the clinicians to provide good care yet respect the patient's right to make decisions. The Oncology and Psychiatry teams struggled with allowing this tumor to progress and take his life without the patient understanding the consequences of his decisions. The natural progression of this tumor would have caused significant misery for the patient before taking his life; therefore, the Oncology team strongly recommended proceeding with surgery and ideally adjuvant radiation.

As is often the case, nurses make unique connections with patients. They have unique perspectives and important insights to patient care. It took several days for the conversation and decision making to evolve. During this time the nursing staff provided excellent care and became endeared to the patient. His voice saying no to surgery was loud and clear to the nursing staff. This created some tension between the physician staff and the nursing staff. Both tried to be respectful, but both groups felt their approach was the best for the patient.

The psychiatry team during this admission deemed the patient unable to make decisions for himself. This was completely different from the assessment made a couple of years ago. We struggled to understand the balance of how to respect individual rights with potentially withholding the basic care that any sound-minded individual would accept and want. Patients with mental health diseases create a unique challenge. This case was scary because we wanted to be sure that we protected the rights of a patient with a mental health disorder while also providing the standard of care to the patient and not depriving him of care. These two goals seemed to be opposing, and it was very unclear how to rectify them and identify the right path.

Last, this case was scary because we did not know who this man was. The police approached the medical team and requested the patient be fingerprinted to assist with identification of the patient. As we contemplated performing a major surgical procedure on a patient with a mental health disease, we wondered what his reaction might be following the surgical procedure. The physicians caring for this patient also knew of a colleague in our community who was recently killed by a patient with mental health illness. Unfortunately, this is a well-known story for physicians. There are stories such as this in many communities across the country. This added a different aspect to the scary nature of this case. We wondered if operating on this patient would be a safety risk for the care team. Yet, we also wondered if denying this patient the standard of care might also someday lead to a dangerous situation.

After days of deliberation among a unique multidisciplinary team we elected to proceed with surgery. The court-appointed legal guardian provided the consent. Surgery was uneventful. He underwent a wide local excision of the skin lesion encompassing the approximately 15 cm in diameter lesion. The deep extent of the resection required removal of the underlying zygoma and temporalis muscle. The frontal branch of the facial nerve was dissected into the parotid and a clear proximal margin was achieved without having to resect any additional facial nerve branches. Parotidectomy and selective dissection were also performed to complete the lymphadenectomy. The defect required a significant reconstruction. We contemplated a wide range of reconstructions varying from simple skin grafting to free flap reconstruction. For this type of defect, a free flap would routinely be used. However, we were concerned about creating any donor site morbidity given the patient's strong desire to avoid surgery. Yet a simple skin graft would have been cosmetically suboptimal and carry a reasonable risk of wound healing problems. We also worried about having a poor cosmetic outcome given the uncertainty of how the patient would respond postoperatively. We ultimately decided to perform a large rotation flap that closed 80% of the defect. The remaining defect was skin grafted. We felt this provided the right balance of cosmetic outcome and optimizing healing while not introducing additional donor site morbidity.

WHAT I LEARNED FROM THIS CASE

What I learned from this case is the importance of respecting individual rights as a patient and team members' opinions. Trying to find the right balance for protecting the rights of a patient with mental illness and trying to ensure the patient is not deprived of the care everyone deserves was very difficult. It was very helpful in this case to begin by identifying key decision points and which decisions could easily be made.

The first step was defining the standard of care for this type of cancer. In this case multidisciplinary input was helpful. The team took its time and did not rush into a plan. This was key to be sure that all positions were considered. We also considered all treatment options including palliative treatment options and weighed the benefits of each approach against the limitations and against the natural history of the tumor. This helped us to focus on the best option for the management of this tumor, surgery followed by adjuvant radiation. With this established it allowed the team to focus energy on the more challenging aspects of this case.

I learned that it is important to know your limitations. I am certainly not an expert on mental illness, and in my routine practice I rarely see patients with untreated mental illness. Engaging the psychiatry team was very helpful. They were helpful not just in their recommendations for medical management but also in doctoring. They helped to frame conversations with the patient and guide interactions. They also provided the critical assessment of whether this patient was competent to make decisions. This was critical to what happened to this patient. Once this decision was made it also helped with decision making. Much like defining standard of care for this type of tumor, this decision was critical and helped clarify the way forward. Similarly, I am not part of the Healthcare for Homeless team, and I am not an expert in this area. Working with the physicians, nurses, and social workers who care for these patients was very helpful, not to mention inspiring. They provided valuable guidance and input to help manage this patient.

I learned to trust my instincts and natural desire to do the right thing for any individual. The team members' underlying focus and desire to take good care of this person drove all of our interactions. This created a healthy respect among team members with differing opinions because each person recognized the other was trying to do the best thing for this patient. This helped prevent people with opposing views from becoming embittered and angry, which would have been easy to do. Intuition and management instincts are largely developed by experience. In this case very few people would say they have a large experience with this exact scenario. However, I have a large experience with managing these types of tumors. This meant I also had the best understanding on the team about the natural history of these tumors and what would happen if we chose to do nothing. It was important to acknowledge this experience and share my instincts with the team, even if it put me at the front of the decision, which could have had a very bad outcome.

CASE OUTCOME

The patient recovered from surgery uneventfully. Fortunately, there were no surgical or anesthesia complications. Upon awakening from surgery the patient was surprisingly melancholy. He did not display any anger or disapproval at having been operated on. The nursing staff on the floor was relieved that he had done well. However, they still wondered if it was the right decision. Their doubts were not about whether surgery would be successful but whether it should be done at all. This question may be answered in time for those who did not agree, or perhaps they will always feel it was the wrong choice.

He healed uneventfully and was ultimately discharged to a facility. He did return for a postoperative visit. This visit was a little anxiety provoking when I saw it on my schedule. I wondered if he would come in angry, would he be violent? Did I put my office and clinic nursing staff at risk? He checked in uneventfully. When I saw him he again expressed no anger or disapproval. At the end of our visit he said thank you! I don't think that made the decision right. It was the right decision based on the time and effort we put into making the decision. But it did feel good, as I think he was genuinely grateful. I suspect some of his reluctance to undergo surgery was the same as any sound-minded person—fear. Having gone through surgery and recovered well, there was no fear remaining. Interestingly, at this point postoperatively he was not at all opposed to radiation therapy and willingly underwent treatment completing it without complication or treatment break. He has come back for a few follow-up visits and remains disease free.

Amazingly, through this process his real identity was discovered. Due to his mental illness he had a major falling out with his family several years before. They had been looking for him ever since and were incredibly grateful to know he was alive and well.

CHAPTER 11

Facial Excision

Maintaining Control in the Face of Cancer

Daniel G. Deschler

THE CASE

A simple statement was next to her name on the clinic schedule, "*Female, born 1927. New facial cancers.*" Truly one of the great understatements. The plural form of the word *cancer* should have tipped me off. Jane's past medical history was a bit more complex, and her recollection of the details was a bit blurred. She had a right mid-face malignant fibrous histiosarcoma removed many years ago. The tumor recurred in 1989 and was resected by John Conley, MD, with a right radical maxillectomy, orbital exenteration, and infratemporal fossa resection extending to the middle skull base and the cavernous sinus. After this, she received radiation therapy. Since that time, she had multiple facial and scalp basal cell and squamous cell carcinomas resected including a significant right upper lip resection. She had no other major medical issues.

That day, she presented with lesions she said have been slowly progressive over the previous years. This included a 2.5-cm ulcerative lesion above the right orbit exenteration defect, which was biopsy-proven basal cell carcinoma. The left oral commissure was replaced by a firm, endophytic lesion, measuring 2 × 1.5 cm that was biopsy-proven squamous cell carcinoma. Yet, the dominating lesion was a sclerosing mass that had replaced her entire nose and midface, approaching—but not directly involving—the left medial canthus and orbit of her remaining seeing eye. The pathology of this lesion was aggressive carcinoma with spindle features that could not be further characterized.

Unlike her medical history, her social history was quite straightforward. Jane lived alone on a small farm in a rural New England state. She was accompanied by her supportive, extended family. She did not smoke or use significant amounts of alcohol. Her only medication was levothyroxine, required after undergoing a previous total thyroidectomy for benign disease. Her therapeutic goals entering this clinical encounter were also quite straightforward. She wished to have these tumors completely removed and controlled but was adamant about maintaining the key functions that would allow her to remain living independently. These included the maintenance of her current vision, the ability to speak in an understandable, albeit somewhat altered fashion, and to maintain an oral diet. In the context of this, a thorough discussion was had with the intent of realistically accommodating these goals, while providing appropriate surgical treatment of these three progressive malignancies.

The risks, benefits, and complications were discussed in detail, as were the intraoperative decisions, which might lead to the procedure being aborted. These were primarily related to potential disease extension requiring orbital exenteration or unresectable skull-base involvement. The reconstructive plan would center on the use of microvascular free tissue transfer with a radial forearm flap and judicious split-thickness skin grafting. She agreed to proceed with surgery.

Under general anesthesia, each of the malignancies was further examined in conjunction with appropriate radiographic imaging. As horrific as her disease appeared, there were favorable components to it, which included the central tumor stopping short of the remaining left orbit (Figure 11–1). Likewise, there was no obvious deep extension toward the anterior skull base or central skull base. The central lesion was approached at its interface with the remaining eye and orbit. Appropriate oncologic cuts were made and margins sent. When these returned negative, the decision was made to proceed with resection of the main lesion. The tumor was excised directly with underlying medial maxilla and septum, delivering it in an *en bloc* fashion. Further ethmoidectomy and maxillectomy were completed on the left side and margins were sent circumferentially and deeply. All these returned negative. The oral commissure cancer was resected to clear margin leaving a significant defect at the oral commissure involving both the upper and lower lip (Figure 11–2). The tumor above the right orbit was approached similarly and excised down to the underlying bone and all margins were found to be clear.

The reconstruction was undertaken in a sequential fashion. A split-thickness skin graft was placed at the right superior orbital defect with excellent coverage. With the central defect and the commissure defect remaining, a large radial forearm flap was then harvested from the right arm in the standard fashion (Figure 11–3). As a total nasal reconstruction was not a tenable option for numerous reasons (lack of adequate midface supports, poor quality of the recipient radiated bed, and lack of availability of forehead flaps due to previous and current resections), the intent of the free tissue transfer was to provide soft tissue coverage of the midface defect internally and externally, while also reconstructing the oral commissure in a manner that would limit microstomia and provide adequate function.

Working in a sequential fashion, the distal aspect of the flap was placed providing internal lining. The flap was then folded upon itself with appropriate de-epithelization to provide

76 SCARY CASES IN OTOLARYNGOLOGY

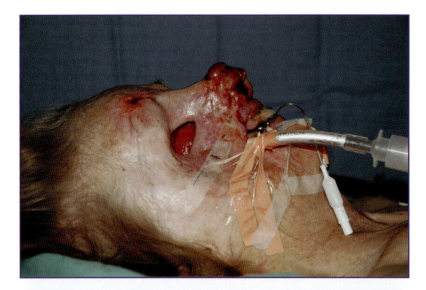

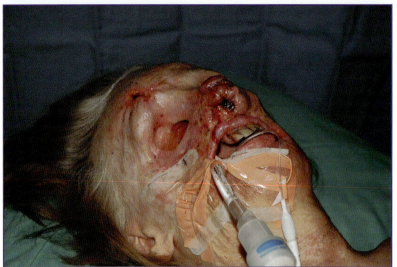

Figure 11–1. Anterior and lateral views demonstrating the three new malignancies: right brow, nasal and midface, and left oral commissure.

external coverage. Further de-epithelialization was then done allowing a separate island on the proximal flap to be folded onto itself to re-create the left oral commissure (Figure 11–4). The pedicle and the vessels were tunneled into the left neck, and the microvascular anastomoses were completed. A tracheotomy was placed as well as a palatal prosthesis, which had been formed prior to the procedure. Her postoperative course was largely uneventful.

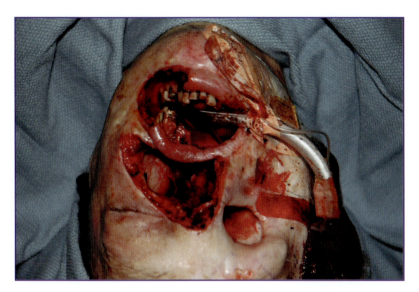

Figure 11–2. Appearance after resection of the three malignancies to clear margins.

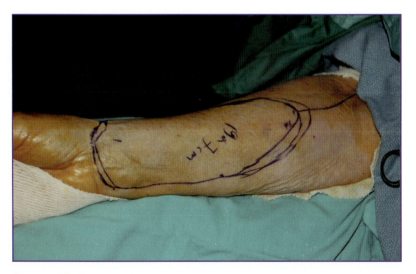

Figure 11–3. Planned harvest of a large radial forearm free flap from the nondominant arm.

During her hospital stay, the tracheotomy tube and the feeding tube were removed and oral alimentation was resumed in conjunction with deglutition therapy. Her major complaint postoperatively consisted of drooling, which she tolerated but found problematic in social situations. She likewise found

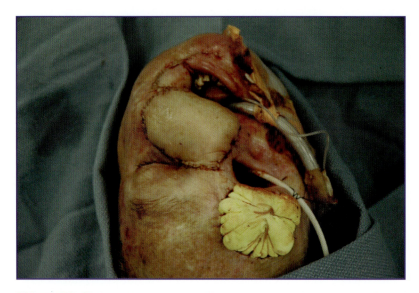

Figure 11–4. Immediate postoperative appearance after reconstruction of the midface and oral commissure defects with the radial forearm free flap and the brow defect with a split-thickness skin graft.

challenge with articulation but maintained acceptably understandable speech.

Jane maintained close clinical follow-up over the ensuing years. A small revision procedure was undertaken to remove some of the redundancy of the central external component of the flap and provide for better competence of the upper lip (Figure 11–5). She also underwent minor adjustments of her palatal prosthesis. She followed closely with her dermatologist who successfully addressed subsequent limited cutaneous cancers. Jane remained fully independent at her home, and the family reveled in her unrelenting desire to mow her own lawn. She kept all her follow-up appointments (Figure 11–6). One day during the summer of 2010, the neighbor noted that Jane's grass had grown a bit longer than usual and asked the police to investigate. They discovered that Jane had passed away in her home of a likely cardiac event, just shy of her 83rd birthday.

Cases such as Jane's can be overwhelming—to the patient, to the family, and to the health care team. The challenges are numerous: previous advanced cancer, deforming surgery and radiation therapy, three new malignancies of varying histologies, no effective nonsurgical treatment, potentially life-prolonging surgery but only with significant attendant morbidity,

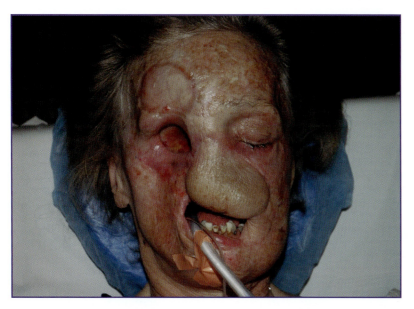

Figure 11–5. Appearance 9 months postoperatively at time of revision to decrease bulk at the upper lip.

and specific functional goals expressed by the patient in addition to her desire to have her disease "cured." For these reasons and more, one could consider this a *"scary case."*

Yet, if we break the situation down by asking a set of specific, binary questions (yes/no) questions in a clear sequence, we can begin to formulate a clear and effective plan. The answers to the questions are based on the available data such as clinical history, physical exam, scans, and pathology as well as upon the patient's clearly stated goals—medical and functional.

Question 1: *Is the disease resectable?*
Answer 1: Yes

Question 2: *Can each lesion be controlled and potentially cured with surgical treatment?*
Answer 2: Yes. Jane's disease had no obvious features making it unresectable (carotid encasement, deep neck fascial involvement, etc). She also had no evidence of metastatic disease.

Question 3: *Will she realistically maintain functions of critical importance to her described quality of life—sight, deglutition, speech?*
Answer 3: Yes

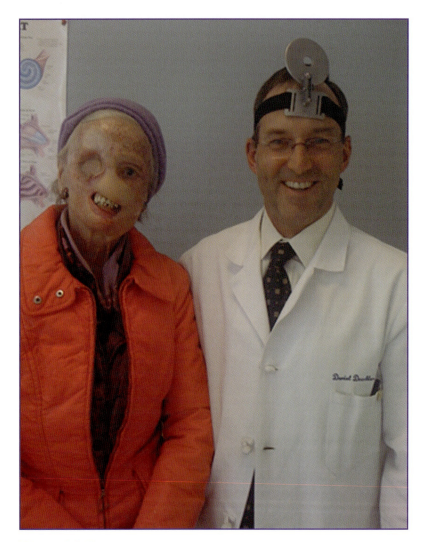

Figure 11–6. Appearance 3½ years postoperatively at routine follow-up visit while still living self-sufficiently in rural New England.

Question 4: *If disease extent intraoperatively required extension of the procedure to adjoining areas, such as the orbit, would she wish to proceed?*
Answer 4: No. Under no circumstances did Jane wish her remaining eye to be removed. Therefore, the ablative approach to the tumor encroaching on the remaining eye would begin by first assessing the ability to remove the disease while preserving the eye. If the disease required orbital exenteration or vision impairment, the procedure would be aborted.

> ***Question 5:*** *Is Jane's expectation to have cosmetic facial appearance return to the state before these cancers and even better? Did she expect to have a "new nose" reconstructed?*
> ***Answer 5:*** No and No. Jane had a realistic expectation of what reconstruction can achieve and how it relates to her overall disease process. She desired functional success over cosmetic.

With these straightforward questions answered, an appropriate ablative plan was made with discrete decision points along the way:

1. Examine under anesthesia to ensure resectability.
2. Explore the aggressive midface mass as it abutted the remaining eye. Send appropriate margins.
3. If margins at eye are clear, proceed with midface resection. Send margins.
4. Proceed to resection of oral commissure lesion. Send margins.
5. Resect the least aggressive cancer at the orbital exenteration defect rim and send margins.
6. While awaiting margins, complete left neck dissection and vessel dissection for later microvascular re-anastomosis.
7. Harvest a large, single paddled radial forearm flap from the right (nondominant arm). Flap size should be larger than the exact measurements of the defects to allow for flexibility in reconstruction of each defect.
8. When margins clear, begin reconstruction, with the originally stated reconstructive goals in mind: preserve eye function, allow for acceptable deglutition and speech rehabilitation. The forearm flap is extremely versatile and can be folded and de-epithelialized after harvest and as the flap is being inset to assure that optimal positioning is achieved. A large initial size of the flap facilitates this.
9. Split-thickness skin grafts are used for the brow lesion and the radial forearm donor site.

In short order, by asking and answering a few appropriate questions, a concise and clear operative plan was formed. Jane's case proceeded as planned with favorable intraoperative findings and acceptable long-term results—far from perfect—but acceptable (Table 11–1).

Table 11–1. Treatment Goals		Yes	No
Tumor Clearance			
	Midface	x	
	Brow	x	
	Oral Commissure	x	
Maximize Function			
	Vision	x	
	Deglutination	x	
	Speech	x	
Cosmesis			x

THIS CASE WAS SCARY BECAUSE

Jane's case was not *scary* because of her appearance on presentation, and it was not *scary* because of the post-op appearance with which she was left. For anything to be truly "scary," there must be an element of fear. The core of such fear usually directly relates to a loss of control. To be functional caregivers, we need to regain some control of the situation and corral the "scary" elements. This was done by acquiring the available data, having Jane articulate her wishes, asking and answering a small set of pertinent questions, and formulating a clear plan. This plan returned control to Jane and to her caregivers in the setting of a somewhat overwhelming clinical presentation.

The truly scary element of Jane's case, that which threatened control for Jane and her caregivers, was the progressive, unrelenting, and unforgiving nature of her malignant disease, which exposed not only our basic human frailty, but the limitations of our current therapeutics. John Conley, MD, Jane's previous surgeon and a pioneer in head and neck cancer surgery, stated this well in the introduction to his book, *Concepts in Head and Neck Surgery:* "An effort has been made to correlate the essentiality of recognizing that major ablative surgery in the head and neck causes crippling of many of the essential physiologic functions in this region and frequently establishes a significant mutilation. This combination of effects has controlled the surgical principles in management."[1] Jane knew this. She had a clear idea of how much function and life quality she would allow to be sacrificed in battling her disease. Our greatest challenge was to listen and respect her wishes. Jane never let fear of her disease and its consequences dominate her, nor should we, as we bring our limited tools to bear against such unrelenting disease. The strength of the human spirit revealed by Jane as she battled her disease makes the story of Jane more *inspiring* than scary.

REFERENCE

1. Conley J. Introduction. In: Conley J, ed. *Concepts in Head and Neck Surgery*. New York, NY: Grune & Stratton; 1970: VII.

CHAPTER 12

Unrelenting Ménière Disease

Ear Surgery in an Only Hearing Ear

Daniel J. Lee
Samuel R. Barber

THE CASE

JC is an otherwise healthy man who at age 35 years presented to the Mass Eye and Ear Otology clinic with a chief complaint of left ear fullness, hearing loss, and vertigo for about a month and a half. He reported similar symptoms in his right ear during his late 20s that was diagnosed as Ménière disease. As a result, he had a right-sided labyrinthectomy at age 31 that cured his dizziness but left him with profound hearing loss of the right ear.

JC had hoped that his episodic dizziness would never return, but unfortunately he reported that his vertigo had returned to the point that he had chronic nausea and intermittent vomiting. He had followed a conservative treatment plan for Ménière disease by adhering to a strict low-salt diet. An updated audiogram showed sensorineural hearing loss with a pure-tone average of 38 dB in his only hearing left ear. He also attempted a trial of diuretics but returned to the clinic 1 month later with progressive balance and hearing issues.

Despite 3 rounds of intratympanic injections of dexamethasone solution to the newly affected left ear, JC's condition only worsened. He experienced 6 severe vertigo attacks in 1 month's time, and his downsloping audiogram showed persistent hearing loss (Figure 12–1). With the combined symptoms of recurrent vertigo attacks, aural fullness, tinnitus, and hearing loss that fluctuated in the low frequencies, JC had all the classic features for Ménière disease involving his only hearing ear.

Between failed conservative therapies and worsening symptoms with disabling vertigo attacks, the decision was made for JC to undergo another surgery on his only hearing ear to address his dizziness. Reasonable options in light of JC's situation were surgical procedures that offered the possibility of both reducing his vestibular symptoms and preserving residual hearing. Intratympanic gentamicin was not a palatable option for the patient, even with acceptable hearing preservation rates in patients with Ménière disease. In the end, a very emotional JC and family were given the options of observation, intratympanic gentamicin, transmastoid endolymphatic sac decompression, or a more invasive retrosigmoid craniotomy with vestibular nerve section.

After much deliberation JC elected to proceed with a canal up mastoidectomy and endolymphatic sac decompression. The surgery went well without any complications, but unfortunately, the procedure did not help alleviate any of his symptoms of dizziness. One week after surgery, JC reported

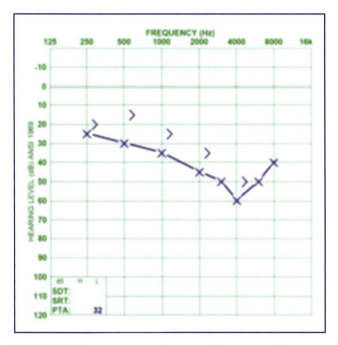

Figure 12–1. Audiogram in August 2008 showed downsloping sensorineural hearing loss on the left side (right ear thresholds not shown due to known history of anacusis). The patient had failed 3 rounds of intratympanic (IT) dexamethasone therapy and continued to have disabling vertigo attacks alongside diminished hearing.

fluctuating hearing loss and daily attacks of vertigo. In addition to dealing with postoperative pain that was poorly controlled with standard prescriptions for narcotic medications, JC was severely distressed that his only hearing had worsened after surgery. JC required reassurance that his hearing would improve with resolution of his hemotympanum.

Over a month later, JC experienced 22 attacks of vertigo. These attacks lasted 2 to 4 hours, and were accompanied by nausea, vomiting, fluctuating hearing loss, and tinnitus that aggravated a persistent baseline level of dizziness and postoperative pain. On the upside, his hearing improved somewhat. A follow-up audiogram showed 30 to 40 dB bone curve with a small air-bone gap. As a former electrician who was unable to work due to his disabling condition, his own "electrical wiring" of the peripheral auditory system, so to speak, had ironically gone awry.

JC's condition was quickly evolving into a scary case for the patient, family, and caregivers. He had worsening symptoms in the only hearing ear and management options to improve his debilitating vertigo could cause (1) deafness and (2) chronic gait instability and oscillopsia. JC was offered intratympanic gentamicin but was understandably reluctant due to concerns of ototoxicity.

After much deliberation, JC elected to pursue a definitive surgical treatment plan for his vertigo attacks that would theoretically preserve residual hearing. A left-sided posterior fossa craniotomy and vestibular neurectomy was that option, but hearing preservation was not guaranteed, and this surgery would commit this patient to bilateral vestibular hypofunction and chronic gait instability. Was this a fate worse than vertigo attacks? Ultimately, JC was fully prepared to lose all of his residual hearing if complications occurred and understood the possibility of needing yet another surgery to place a cochlear implant. After completing both neurotologic and neurosurgical evaluations, JC and his family decided together that a retrosigmoid approach was best, and the vestibular nerve would be identified and selectively cut within the cerebellopontine angle. A long discussion about the risks of hearing loss and facial nerve palsy, in addition to the possibility of a postcraniotomy headache and cerebrospinal fluid (CSF) leak, took place. Continuous neuromonitoring with auditory brainstem responses was requested to monitor the integrity of his auditory pathways surgery.

Surgery was challenging. JC's soft demeanor was offset by a large body habitus, prominent shoulders, and short neck. Completion of the craniotomy and exposure of the cranial nerves was exceedingly difficult, with the surgeons' arms and hands fully stretched to even reach the 7th/8th nerve complex. Microinstruments were held by the fingertips to reach the neural anatomy and dissect the plane between the cochlear and vestibular branches of the 8th cranial nerve and to sharply divide the vestibular nerve. Fortunately, there was no threshold shift or loss of morphology seen on brainstem evoked auditory responses and facial electromyograms (EMGs) remained quiet. He had an uncomplicated hospital stay.

After vestibular nerve sectioning JC did not initially experience a single recurrent violent episode of dizziness or vertigo, about which he was quite pleased. At his first postoperative follow-up visit, he did report a slight decrease in hearing. He noticed this change after completing the oral steroid taper following his hospital discharge. He was put on oral steroids again for a month, but his hearing did not improve.

JC enjoyed a total of 4 months without any episodic dizziness or vertigo following surgery. Much to everyone's dismay, however, mild symptoms began to manifest once again. JC counted 12 episodes of vertigo this time, but none of these were quite as debilitating as before. This was an exceptionally tumultuous clinical course of bilateral intractable Ménière disease involving multiple surgeries, right-sided deafness, craniotomy surgery, and now recurrent vertigo attacks associated with the left ear. JC was prepared to sacrifice all of his hearing in order to definitively end his relentless problems with vertigo and dizziness.

JC was now willing to undergo gentamicin therapy in his only hearing ear to chemically ablate any remaining aberrant vestibular hair cell activity. The major risk of a chemical labyrinthectomy, although small, would be permanent deafness. The first round of gentamicin resulted in temporarily relief, so two more rounds were administered. JC's residual hearing was indeed preserved; however, the dizziness did not go away. As such, JC then underwent surgery again for this left ear, a transcanal middle ear exploration with placement of gentamicin pledgets directly upon the round and oval windows. During this procedure, a pseudomembrane was discovered over the round window, which was subsequently removed to facilitate better absorption of gentamicin into the inner ear.

JC still had vertiginous symptoms and worsening sensorineural hearing loss in the left ear despite exhaustive medical and surgical interventions with a goal of hearing conservation. To further evaluate JC's vestibular function, additional testing was performed. Cold caloric testing showed absent responses bilaterally, but surprisingly there were normal cervical vestibular evoked myogenic potentials (cVEMPs) in the left ear. This suggested residual vestibular function and a functioning saccule and inferior vestibular nerve on the left side. JC was potentially a candidate for cochlear implantation, yet a revision vestibular neurectomy might resolve symptoms while preserving residual hearing. After much deliberation among the patient, family, and surgical team, the decision was made to consider a revision craniotomy, decompression of the internal auditory canal (not done at first surgery due to risks of postsurgical headaches from dispersion of bone dust) and vestibular nerve sectioning within the internal auditory canal (IAC). A preoperative magnetic resonance image (MRI) is seen in Figure 12–2.

This revision surgery proved to be a much more challenging procedure as compared to the first vestibular neurectomy. First, although JC lost a substantial amount of weight prior to this operation, surgical access to his posterior fossa was still difficult. Second, he was found to have an anterior inferior cerebellar artery coursing into the internal acoustic

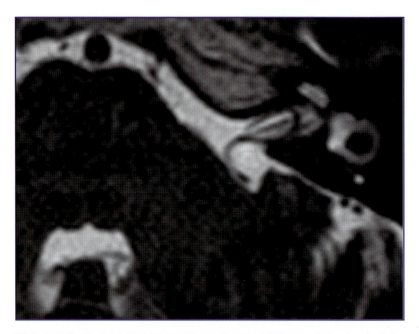

Figure 12–2. Axial MRI T2 3D Fiesta imaging, left ear, at the level of the internal auditory canal (IAC). This pre-craniotomy scan revealed a tortuous anterior inferior cerebellar artery coursing around the 7th to 8th cranial nerve complex within the IAC. This vascular loop added to the complexity of decompressing the IAC to transect the remaining vestibular nerves during his revision posterior fossa craniotomy.

meatus that made drilling treacherous. Third, when the dural was open in the IAC, this same artery was found intertwining between the vestibular and cochlear nerve fibers. Finally, during sectioning of the inferior and superior vestibular nerve fibers, an unfortunate shift in the auditory brainstem response thresholds occurred. The surgical team was encouraged that the vestibular nerve was completely severed during surgery but very concerned about his drop in hearing.

Although there were no complications in the immediate postoperative period, JC soon experienced progressive headaches that became excruciating in character. Initially the surgical team felt that these headaches might have been due to the bone dust contamination that is unavoidable during decompression of the IAC. These headaches can arise after posterior fossa surgery involving bony drilling even if there is careful placement of Gelfoam pledgets before drilling to reduce widespread dispersion of bone dust and meticulous irrigation and débridement of bone dust prior to completion of surgery. However, his symptoms worsened, and he was readmitted to the neurosurgical service for a workup and imaging. A computed tomography (CT) scan showed postsurgical changes (Figure 12–3), and during his hospital stay he was found to have purulent drainage from his craniotomy incision site. He was taken emergently to the operating room for irrigation and drainage of the craniotomy site. A large abscess was evacuated from the epidural and subdural spaces.

The risk of infection was well known to both JC and the surgical team prior to the revision vestibular neurectomy, yet no one was expecting a postoperative course this complicated. JC's condition became increasingly more life threatening over time. One week following his visit to the operating room, he was still draining fluid from his wound. He underwent a

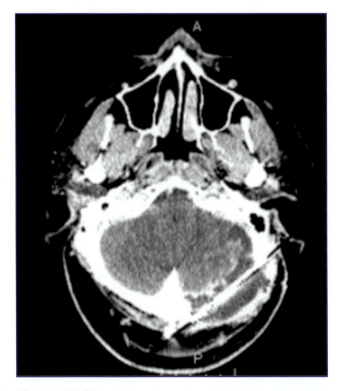

Figure 12–3. Postoperative CT scan taken 2 weeks after left ear revision vestibular neurectomy following revision suboccipital craniotomy approach. A fluid collection along the left cerebellar hemisphere extending superficial to the titanium mesh was seen, including surrounding soft tissue nodular enhancement. The patent was complaining of headaches with increasing severity. A purulent infection was identified and required incision and drainage and removal of titanium cranioplasty hardware.

second procedure that involved the evacuation of a recurrent wound abscess, along with repair of a CSF leak and right frontal ventriculostomy. Thankfully, JC did not encounter any further infections or drainage from the incision site.

Six months later, his symptoms of vertigo were vastly improved with mild, occasional episodes. He did have chronic instability with walking, and reported persistent oscillopsia that required ambulation with a cane. His residual hearing had been stable throughout, albeit usable only with a hearing aid. JC's word recognition, however, was deteriorating compared to prior exams despite having stable thresholds on his audiogram. With JC's left ear vestibular issues now stable, the discussion was begun to determine ways in which JC's quality of life could be optimized by enhancing auditory perception.

After further consultation, JC elected to proceed with a right-sided cochlear implant on the side with the history of prior transmastoid labyrinthectomy. His left ear had residual hearing aided with amplification. JC's hearing was completely gone in the right ear following surgery for his first case of Ménière disease. Thankfully, both CT and MRI demonstrated a fluid-filled normal appearing cochlea despite the prior labyrinthectomy, making JC a reasonable candidate for cochlear implantation. The benefits of "bimodal" hearing (right ear with bionic hearing and left ear with acoustic hearing amplified with a hearing aid) were carefully presented to JC and family.

JC underwent uneventful cochlear implantation on the right side where a prior mastoidectomy and labyrinthectomy were performed. There were no complications during or after the surgery. He did well postoperatively, and following device activation he was found to have behavioral thresholds of 35 dB with his new implant (Figure 12–4). He still struggles with oscillopsia and some instability when walking, but no longer did he suffer from unpredictable and intractable vertigo. After a most difficult and frustrating journey, JC has finally resumed life with drastically reduced dizziness and improved hearing.

MÉNIÈRE DISEASE

Ménière disease is a chronic condition of the inner ear that can affect both the auditory and vestibular pathways. Hallmark symptoms include episodic vertigo attacks, fluctuating hearing loss, aural fullness, and tinnitus. The prevalence of this disease has been reported with high variability, ranging from 200 to 500 per 100,000 persons.[1,2]

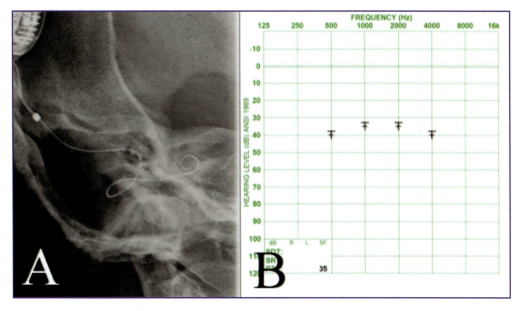

Figure 12–4. A. Reverse Stenvers x-ray view of the mastoid, right ear, shows implant electrode coiled 360 degrees in the expected location of the cochlea. **B.** Postactivation behavioral threshold audiogram demonstrates a pure-tone average of 35 dB in the implanted ear.

The majority of Ménière patients experience unilateral signs and symptoms, while bilateral Ménière disease is found in only 10%.[3] However, over the course of a few decades, 40% to 50% of unilateral Ménière patients will go on to develop bilateral disease. The peak incidence occurs between 30 and 60 years of age, but cases have been described in young children and the elderly.[4,5]

Treatment of Ménière disease depends on the progression of cochlear and vestibular manifestations. Symptoms are episodic in nature, but stabilization of symptoms over time is common. For patients in whom symptoms do not stabilize, most are managed medically. Conservative measures include a restricted salt diet and vestibular rehabilitation. First-line medical therapies include a trial of diuretics, followed by intratympanic steroid injections and short courses of oral steroids.[6,7]

A minority of patients with Ménière disease requires surgical intervention. The most common surgery for patients with persistent symptoms despite medical therapy is an endolymphatic sac decompression.[8] If this procedure does not provide relief for intractable dizziness and vertigo, vestibular ablative techniques are offered. Two surgical procedures for vestibular ablation include vestibular neurectomy performed during a retrosigmoid craniotomy approach (in which the vestibular division of the 8th cranial nerve is sectioned to preserve residual hearing) and transmastoid labyrinthectomy (hearing is sacrificed in this case to surgically ablate vestibular end-organs).[2] An alternative to a surgical approach under general anesthesia is a chemical labyrinthectomy performed in the office setting. A topically anesthetic (typically phenol) is applied to the posteroinferior quadrant of the tympanic membrane and a 25-gauge syringe needle is used to deliver a 40 mg/cc solution of gentamicin into the middle ear. Uptake of gentamicin takes place via the round and oval windows to enter the inner ear fluids. This procedure has been shown to be preferentially vestibulotoxic versus ototoxic with a 20% to 30% risk of worsening hearing; there is clearly a risk of permanent damage to cochlear pathways and subsequent sensorineural hearing loss with inner ear exposure to aminoglycosides.[1,9,10] Hearing conservation is the goal for most approaches for treatment, but patients need to be counseled carefully as any "hearing preservation" approach to treat Ménière disease may result in permanent hearing deficits.[2,9]

The potential morbidity from bilateral Ménière is much more significant. Progressive hearing loss can lead to total deafness in both ears, while a complete lack of vestibular function results in chronic oscillopsia and gait disturbance.[11] One recent advance in technology that may benefit patients with bilateral vestibular dysfunction in the future is the vestibular implant. Electrodes are surgically placed into the individual semicircular canals to electrically stimulate the ampullary nerves using a transmastoid approach. This device is under development at several research institutions internationally, including the University of Geneva in Switzerland, Massachusetts Eye and Ear Infirmary, and Johns Hopkins.[12-14]

Although the worst-case scenario of bilateral Ménière disease is exceedingly rare, any intervention needs to be thoughtfully considered in patients with only one functional ear given the potential for bilateral hearing and vestibular loss. JC was the most severe bilateral Ménière case from our surgical practice in recent history, with disabling vertigo attacks and progressive hearing deterioration refractory to conservative medical and surgical intervention.

THIS CASE WAS SCARY BECAUSE

The majority of patients who experience Ménière disease do not progress to a level of severity or bilaterality that would warrant chronicling as a scary case. JC's story is exceedingly uncommon, and his case of severe bilateral Ménière disease is undoubtedly a rare entity. What started as a classic presentation Ménière in his right ear progressed into increasingly complex pathology bilaterally with life-threatening complications and devastating morbidity. Despite conservative measures and exhaustive efforts to conserve hearing, JC's disabling vertigo persisted while hearing in his only good ear declined insidiously. Every intervention was met with cautious optimism and suspense. The fact that JC's only hearing ear underwent several invasive procedures stands on its own to be deemed a scary case. The occurrence of recurrent intracranial wound abscesses and a CSF leak on the side with progressive sensorineural hearing loss is truly the apotheosis of a scary case. JC's story stands out among many challenging cases in our neurotologic surgical practice at Massachusetts Eye and Ear Infirmary as a very scary case despite an unassuming primary diagnosis at initial presentation.

WHAT I LEARNED FROM THIS CASE

- Ménière disease in an only hearing ear is a challenging problem.
- Conservative measures should be followed if possible.
- Listen to your patient!
  - Is control of vertigo more important than preservation of hearing?
- Use caloric testing and cervical vestibular evoked myogenic potential (cVEMP) testing to assess for residual vestibular function before and after intervention.
- The management plan of the complex Ménière disease patient should follow a multidisciplinary approach with Otology and Neurotology/Otoneurology/Neurosurgery/Audiology/Physical Therapy.
- Maintain open lines of communication with patient and family.

REFERENCES

1. Minor LB, Schessel DA, Carey JP. Ménière's disease. *Curr Opin Neuro*. 2004;17:9–16.
2. Sajjadi H, Paparella MM. Ménière's disease. *Lancet*. 2008;372:406–414.

3. Kitahara M. Bilateral aspects of Ménière's disease. Ménière's disease with bilateral fluctuant hearing loss. *Acta Oto-laryngol Suppl.* 1991;485:74–77.
4. Paparella MM. Pathogenesis and pathophysiology of Ménière's disease. *Acta Oto-laryngol Suppl.* 1991;485:26–35.
5. Alexander TH, Harris JP. Current epidemiology of Ménière's syndrome. *Otolaryngol Clin North Am.* 2010;43: 965–970.
6. Rauch SD. Clinical hints and precipitating factors in patients suffering from Ménière's disease. *Otolaryngol Clin North Am.* 2010;43:1011–1017.
7. Martin Gonzalez C, Gonzalez FM, Trinidad A, et al. Medical management of Ménière's disease: a 10-year case series and review of literature. *Eur Arch of Oto-rhino-laryngol.* 2010; 267:1371–1376.
8. Paparella MM. Endolymphatic sac revision for recurrent intractable Ménière's disease. *Otolaryngol Clin North Am.* 2006;39:713–721, vi.
9. Tassinari M, Mandrioli D, Gaggioli N, Roberti di Sarsina P. Ménière's disease treatment: a patient-centered systematic review. *Audiol Neuro-otol.* 2015;20:153–165.
10. Huon LK, Fang TY, Wang PC. Outcomes of intratympanic gentamicin injection to treat Ménière's disease. *Otol Neurotol.* 2012;33:706–714.
11. Nabi S, Parnes LS. Bilateral Ménière's disease. *Cur Opin Otolaryngol Head Neck Surg.* 2009;17:356–362.
12. Guyot JP, Perez Fornos A, Guinand N, van de Berg R, Stokroos R, Kingma H. Vestibular assistance systems: promises and challenges. *J of Neurol.* 2016;263 Suppl 1:30–35.
13. Merfeld DM, Lewis RF. Replacing semicircular canal function with a vestibular implant. *Cur Opin Otolaryngol Head Neck Surg.* 2012;20:386–392.
14. Fridman GY, Della Santina CC. Progress toward development of a multichannel vestibular prosthesis for treatment of bilateral vestibular deficiency. *Anat Rec* (Hoboken, NJ: 2007). 2012;295:2010–2029.

CHAPTER 13

Unexpected Lymphoma

The Routine Scary Case

Jerry M. Schreibstein

THE CASE

I first met a 22-year-old female aerobics instructor who presented for hoarseness, throat clearing, mild adenopathy, and postnasal drip. She had a history of allergic rhinitis, nasal trauma, and recreational singing. Examination revealed a normal larynx, normal neck lymph nodes, a septal deviation to the right side, and moderate inferior turbinate hypertrophy. She was treated with voice care, allergy medications, and follow-up as needed.

She returned 9 years later for newer problems. She was 31-years-old and had just delivered her second set of twins! Her problems consisted of chronic nasal congestion and postnasal drip. She reported mold exposure at home and had been treated for 6 sinus infections with antibiotics in the last year. Examination revealed bilateral choncha bullosa and a severe septal deviation. I recommended resuming intranasal steroids, saline lavages, and an allergy evaluation. We also discussed possible septoplasty and turbinate reduction. She was too busy with the birth of her twins and opening a new aerobics studio to consider allergic testing or surgical intervention. I treated her with clarithromycin, prednisone, and nasal saline lavage. In vitro allergy testing was ordered as well as a computed tomography (CT) scan of the sinuses in 4 weeks at the time of follow-up visit.

One month later, the allergy testing was negative, she could not tolerate the antibiotics, and prednisone provided very temporary relief. She was also complaining of headache, neck pain, and eye pressure which she attributed to eating Chinese food on the night prior triggering a migraine. The infections were impairing her quality of life with the 4 young children. CT scan was obtained showed minimal sinus disease (Figure 13–1) with septal deviation and concha bullosa. She was busy with her aerobics studio and the 4 kids.

WHAT WOULD YOU DO?

Surgery? More medical therapies? Further allergy workup? My initial thoughts were that she has a long history of quality of life–impairing diseases: allergic rhinitis, recurrent sinusitis, septal deviation, migraine headaches. For quality-of-life disorders, patients usually decide how aggressively to treat symptoms. She declined any additional workup or surgical management.

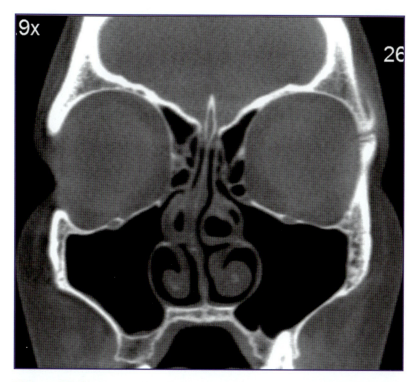

Figure 13–1. CT scan of the sinuses revealed minimal mucosal thickening in the osteomeatal complex, septal deviation to the right side, and bilateral concha bullosa.

She returned 1 year later reporting recurrent episodes of severe facial pain, nasal congestion, and headache. She was having significant work stress and sleep deprivation with the children. She had been treated with 10 courses of antibiotics and multiple 3- to 5-day bursts of prednisone through her primary care provider's office which provided temporary relief. Nasal endoscopy showed a small left middle polyp, which was consistent with progression of her sinus infections. Repeat CT scan of the sinuses revealed ethmoid mucosal edema, worse on the left side and osteomeatal complex obstruction (Figure 13–2).

NOW WHAT?

More antibiotics? Steroids? Observation? Surgery? She even discussed the possibility of seeing a naturopathic provider. The dilemma with routine, quality-of-life diseases, is that when symptoms persist and become atypical, it can be difficult to

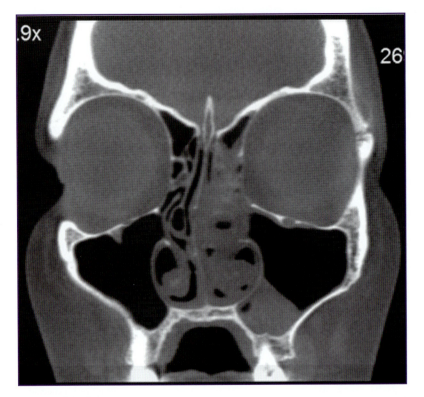

Figure 13–2. Repeat CT scan of the sinuses revealed ethmoid mucosal edema, worse on the left side, and osteomeatal complex obstruction.

push a patient to surgery. She was opening a new studio in 3 weeks. I have had a more than 10-year relationship as her physician and watched her grow up and become a mother of 4. The thought of a complication was scary, but I thought that her symptoms were severe enough to warrant surgery. She finally agreed to nasal and sinus surgery with the understanding that if things go well, she would be able to resume aerobics in 2 weeks.

THE SURGERY

She underwent an uncomplicated bilateral endoscopic ethmoidectomy, maxillary antrostomy with septoplasty and turbinate reduction. There was purulent drainage in the left maxillary sinus with typical appearing polyps and mild mucosal edema (Figure 13–3A). Once the diseased tissue was removed, the sinuses appeared unremarkable (Figure 13–3B). Nothing scary happened!

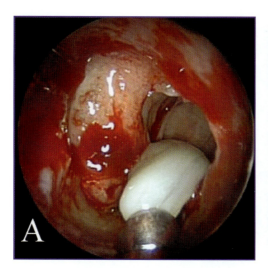
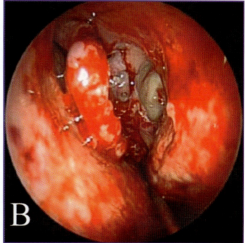

Figure 13–3. A. Endoscopic view during left ethmoidectomy and maxillary antrostomy. There was purulent drainage in the left maxillary sinus with typical appearing polyps and mild mucosal edema. **B.** Once the polyps were removed, the sinus mucosa appeared unremarkable.

She returned for splint removal on postoperative day 4 and pathology was still pending, but not unusual for a late afternoon Thursday case. The pathologist called (never a good sign) to say that he was concerned about a predominance of small lymphocytes and extensive inflammation suggestive for lymphoma (Figure 13–4). In disbelief, I report that nothing seemed out of the ordinary given the recurrent acute infectious history and chronic sinus disease. I could not imagine that a routine sinus surgery found a lymphoma.

HOW DO YOU DELIVER THIS NEWS?

The patient required lots of handholding postoperatively with complaints of nasal irritation, headaches, and anxiety about opening a new business. I could not have a discussion over the phone. Additionally, I was holding out hope that the pathologist was wrong. She returned on post-op day 10 for removal of an intranasal suture that was causing irritation. I had to inform her of the pending pathology since additional tissue was necessary for flow cytometry to confirm the diagnosis. She responded, "I have 4 kids, am I going to die? I feel fine, something must be wrong."

Additional tissue confirmed an aggressive natural killer cell lymphoma (EBV positive). She had second and third opinions,

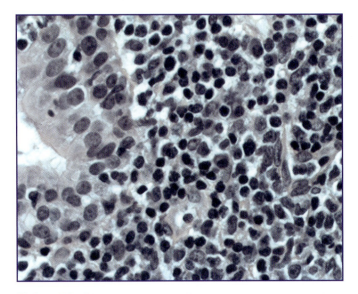

Figure 13–4. High-power view of the pathologic specimen from the left sinus surgery. There is a predominance of small lymphocytes suggestive for lymphoma which turned out to be an aggressive natural killer cell lymphoma on flow cytometry.

extensive workup that included bone marrow biopsy, positron emission tomography (PET)/CT, and additional blood and tissue specimens.

THIS CASE WAS SCARY BECAUSE

- A 31-year-old mother of 4 children with a malignancy is scary!
- It is difficult to deal with an unexpected diagnosis for both the patient and the surgeon. How does a physician stay mostly composed when delivering bad news to a long-term patient? Dr. Itzak Brook suggested to us at the American Academy of Otolaryngology-Head and Neck Surgery (AAO-HNS) annual meeting that it is okay to hug a patient, but is it really appropriate? I once learned of a surgeon who cried with his patient when giving a terminal diagnosis and was later sued for delayed diagnosis. The family thought that the surgeon was so upset because he made a mistake.
- I didn't know if I had missed the diagnosis! Were there any signs that could have tipped me off sooner?

- The decision for surgery was scary because the patient had apparent quality-of-life diseases. Is it ever right to push patient into surgery?
- Managing a disease where there are few experts and a poor prognosis is scary when the patient counts on you for information and support.
- Natural killer cell lymphoma needs a new name. It is not fair to tell patients that they have this diagnosis. No disease should contain the words "natural killer," even though it refers to the cell type rather than the prognosis.

FOLLOW-UP

She underwent extensive chemotherapy, radiation therapy, and stem cell transplant. It was an extremely rocky course, both physically and emotionally for both of us. She sent me e-mails throughout treatment. Through the many ups and downs, we tried to stay focused on a positive outcome. At 1-year post-treatment, she held a fundraiser party for other cancer patients where she embarrassed her surgeon with highlights of his support. She is now 4 years out and has no evidence of disease.

WHAT I LEARNED FROM THIS CASE

The unexpected diagnosis should always be in the back of our mind. We see routine, quality-of-life problems on a regular basis. It is easy to get lulled into the routine of textbook medicine, but we should always be on the lookout for those subtle signs and symptoms that don't exactly fit the diagnosis. I also learned that even diseases with poor prognoses can have good outcomes. Finally, I learned what Itzak Brook had suggested: it is okay to have closer professional relationships with patients who need support. My care for her did not end with the diagnosis as I followed her through treatment and recovery.

CHAPTER 14

Tracheotomy

A Scary Chief Complaint

Bruce R. Gordon

URGENT REFERRAL FROM A COLLEAGUE

Last January I received a call from a trusted General Surgeon colleague, referring a 23-year-old female for an urgent tracheotomy. He said she had a necrotic ulcer overlying her subclavian access port, which had been caused by extravasated epinephrine used to treat anaphylaxis. She had a history of frequent intubations, and tracheotomy had been recommended at another hospital. I agreed to book the earliest day we could both work together in the operating room, and quickly scheduled her office visit.

FIRST OFFICE VISIT

The patient arrived accompanied by her mother, who participated in the interview. Except for the 4-cm necrotic wound on her upper right chest (Figure 14–1), and being somewhat overweight, the young woman appeared to be well. She related a history that was complex and progressively serious. At age 3, she had the onset of intermittent urticaria, treated successfully with antihistamines. But, by age 15, she began to have oropharyngeal and laryngeal edema episodes, often requiring epinephrine treatment, and gradually becoming more frequent.

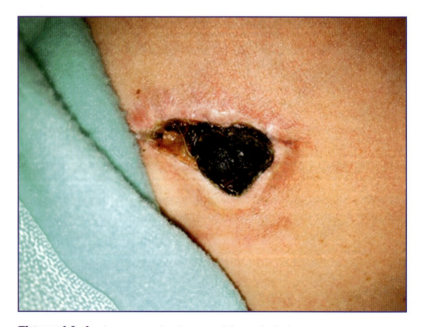

Figure 14–1. 4-cm necrotic ulcer overlying subclavian port.

Currently, she was being intubated about every other month. A subclavian access port had been implanted, and subsequently revised 5 times, to assist in IV epinephrine use during her attacks. She had been treated as an emergency in, or had been referred to, 11 different hospitals in Eastern Massachusetts and Rhode Island (Figure 14–2). She said her symptoms developed rapidly, without any obvious trigger, from an itchy rash to oral edema and then to dyspnea and voice change. She had developed hoarseness after many intubations, and once was nearly aphonic for a month. She fears she will lose her voice. On her last hospitalization, epinephrine extravasated, with resulting necrosis over the upper chest port site. Finally, she said the ear, nose, and throat (ENT) consultant at that hospital advised a tracheotomy.

The past medical history was remarkable for type 1 diabetes since age 16, with an implanted insulin pump placed 2 year ago. She said her glucose levels were unstable due to frequent corticosteroid use. She also had long-standing acid reflux, and had been treated for Lyme disease and ehrlichiosis

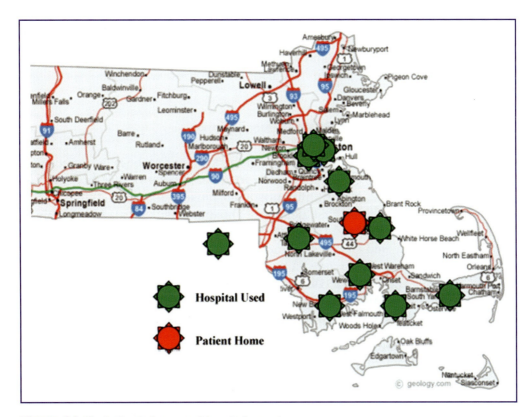

Figure 14–2. Patient's home and hospitals used.

2 years previously. Family history included respiratory allergy, thyroid problems, diabetes, cancer, coronary artery disease, and easy bleeding. Her social history was that she had considered a medical career, and was working as an aid to disabled adults, but she was losing so much time from work because of her medical problems, that she was applying for disability.

She lived at her parents' home, and was exposed to dogs and cats. She had reactions to many antibiotics, diphenhydramine, fexofenadine, hydroxychloroquine, and ondansetron. She had seen an allergist at one of the area's finest medical centers, extensive allergy prick tests were negative, and multiple preventative treatments for idiopathic anaphylaxis were either unsuccessful or were not tolerated.

The physical exam showed a mild breathy hoarseness, a normal head and neck, normal fiberoptic laryngoscopy, and normal skin, except for the 4-cm right upper chest, mobile, necrotic wound.

TREATMENT PLAN

The patient signed record releases for the 11 other hospitals, and I scheduled her for an office pulmonary function test, pre-op labs, and direct laryngoscopy, tracheotomy, and, with General Surgery, excision of the chest wound.

RECORDS REVIEW

Eventually, about a 15-cm-thick pile of records were received, but less than half came in the 2 weeks before her surgery. The 2 community hospitals closest to the patient's home responded first, detailing 2 hospital visits in 2011 and again in 2013. Most lab tests showed normal values, except for changes caused by her treatments. The records stated that the patient had experienced a total of 9 intubations by 2011, 20 by 2013, and 25 by 2014. About a month previously, a new subclavian port was placed under general anesthesia, and in recovery, she had itching and throat symptoms, was re-intubated, and given IV epinephrine, which extravasated. During that visit, she had multiple consultations. The ENT consultant found she was slightly hoarse, had mild arytenoid erythema, and a slight gap on phonation. In order to pinpoint a diagnosis, he recommended endoscopy prior to any future intubation.

The third set of records came from a major medical center, where there were 4 admissions between January 2013 and January 2014, with no documented laryngeal edema, normal pulmonary function tests, and normal upper endoscopy. The respiratory lab technician documented that the patient's voice was normal. Of concern, multiple electrocardiograms showed new ischemia during epinephrine treatments.

The fourth records response, from the closest hospital to the patient's home, showed 12 emergency visits in 2007, 7 in 2008, 5 in 2009, 14 in 2010, including one intubation, 5 in 2011, with 1 incidence of post-op itching, and 6 visits in 2012. Allergy prick tests there were negative, except for weak reactions to dog and cat. In half of these visits there were no visible hives or rash, and in the others, there was no skin exam documented. Finally, 3 physicians noted the patient had both anxiety and a flat affect, and she refused an offered psychiatric evaluation.

After this records review, there was no clear indication for tracheotomy, and many concerns. I scheduled an extra pre-op visit with the patient and her mother, during which I recommended no tracheotomy, but only a laryngoscopy, and wound excision. The patient broke down hysterically sobbing, and pleaded for a tracheotomy. It was now crystal clear that she suffered from Munchausen syndrome.

MUNCHAUSEN SYNDROME

Munchausen syndrome is named after Hieronymus Carl Friedrich Baron von Münchhausen (1720–1797), a German nobleman, and famous teller of tall tales. Classified as a factitious disorder,[1] or a somatic symptom disorder,[2] Munchausen syndrome, and similar ailments, are very common, with an incidence estimated to be greater than 25% of all patients seen in family practices. A typical profile of an identified Munchausen syndrome patient is a female health care worker in young middle age. Symptoms often begin in the teens, but the age at first diagnosis for women is 31, and for men, 39.[3] Patients with Munchausen syndrome doctor shop and have health care costs much higher than average: 6-fold higher for hospitalizations, and 14-fold higher for outpatient services.[4] Disability is common, with 82% stopping work. Common features of Munchausen syndrome include unexplained somatic symptoms, chronicity, social dysfunction, occupational difficulty, increased health care use, and both high patient and physician dissatisfaction with the therapeutic relationship.[5] This patient had evidence for all of these, except for social dysfunction. Munchausen patients show levels or degrees of severity, from presenting a factitious history, to symptom simulation, exaggeration, aggravation, and self-induction of disease. These levels may overlap and change over time.[3] Munchausen syndrome shares features with other somatic symptom disorders, including somatization disorder, conversion disorder, pain disorder, hypochondriasis, factitious disorder by proxy, and malingering.[4] This case shared features of both Munchausen syndrome and Munchausen by proxy, since the mother was highly involved in the patient's care, and the unusual history began in the patient's childhood (Table 14–1).

Treatment of Munchausen syndrome is difficult. Many experts recommend that after establishing the diagnosis, attempts be made to create a strong primary care–patient relationship, and to change the treatment goal from curing to caring. How to "deliver" the diagnosis is controversial, but allowing patients to save face, and meeting the patient's emotional needs, while steering them away from unneeded treatments, is the goal. I did not tell this patient what I suspected, but I did tell her I did not believe she needed a tracheotomy. I explained that her larynx needed a careful direct examination, which had not yet been done, and I agreed to do that. She calmed down, showed up for surgery, and eventually healed well from the wound excision. Her laryngoscopy, of course, was normal, and her vocal cord motion on awakening was also normal.

Table 14–1. Frequency of Types of Evidence Leading to a Diagnosis of Munchausen's Syndrome[1]

Inexplicable test results	45%
History inconsistent or implausible	35%
Visited >3 medical centers for problem	30%
Patient confession	17%
Outside records search	16%
Observed tampering	12%
Hidden medications found	4%
Family revelation	3%

WHAT I LEARNED FROM THIS CASE

Medicine is like diplomacy: trust, but verify. Especially in a complex case, request and review outside records. And, when someone requests your records, send them promptly. Further, do not let the patient direct his or her care over your best judgement. When I was a young surgeon, I made the mistake a few times of letting a patient convince me of what to do, and it was always a big mistake. This case was a cogent reminder of the wisdom of demanding solid indications before performing surgery.

There is another aspect of Munchausen syndrome that needs airing. Once the diagnosis is made, patients still need to have honest and complete evaluation of their complaints, because they can, like any other patient, develop a second, nonpsychiatric disease. Because this patient did have 2 weakly positive prick tests, I thought that she might actually have low sensitivity or non-IgE allergies that were responsible for her skin itching symptoms. She consented to additional allergy testing, which was positive, but as soon as I raised the possibility of curative, safe sublingual allergy treatment, she vanished.

This patient has now moved on to other doctors and other hospitals. She gets cardiac ischemia from epinephrine. She gives a very scary, very convincing history, and she knows her chosen disease well. She doctor shops, and could be anywhere. Who will give her the fatal dose of epinephrine, or operate, and inadvertently cause a fatal complication? In this case, the wound necrosis could have involved the port, causing sepsis, morbidity, and possible mortality. The patient was very fortunate, this time. Yet, an unknown number of Munchausen syndrome patients die every year from unnecessary medical interventions. She, or others like her, will show up in your hospital soon. Will you be prepared?

REFERENCES

1. American Psychiatric Association (APA). *Diagnostic and Statistical Manual of Mental Disorders*. 4th ed, Text rev. Washington, DC: Author; 2000.
2. American Psychiatric Association (APA). *Diagnostic and Statistical Manual of Mental Disorders*. 5th ed. Washington, DC: Author; 2013.

3. Krahn LE, Li H, O'Connor MK. Patients who strive to be ill: factitious disorder with physical symptoms. *Am J Psychiatry*. 2003 Jun;160(6):1163–1168.
4. McCahill M. *Am Fam Phys*. 1995;52:193–203.
5. Sharma MP, Manjula M. Behavioural and psychological management of somatic symptom disorders: an overview. *Int Rev Psychiatry*. 2013 Feb;25(1):116–124.

SECTION 4

Neural Injury

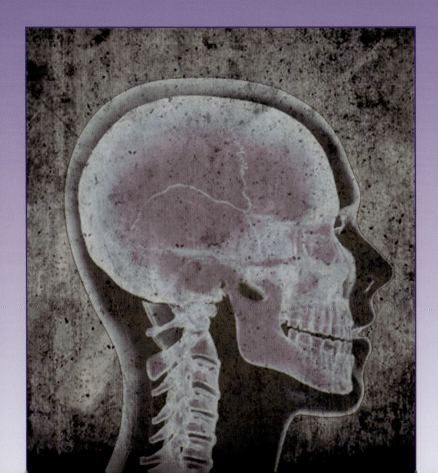

CHAPTER 15

Orbital Hematoma

In the Public Eye

**Ralph Metson
Christopher David Brook**

THE CASE

A 57-year-old pharmacist presented for outpatient evaluation of chronic nasal congestion. He reported a history of sinusitis dating back to childhood, with the development of chronic frontal headaches and maxillary pressure over the last few years. He had undergone endoscopic sinus surgery and septoplasty at another institution 2 years prior. In addition, the patient had undergone allergy testing that demonstrated sensitivity to some common allergens. He was on a maintenance dose of nasal steroids and oral antihistamines. In the year preceding presentation he had taken several courses of antibiotics and oral steroid tapers with only transient relief of his symptoms.

Nasal endoscopy was notable for a septal deviation with mucopurulent discharge and bilateral nasal polyps visible in the middle meatus regions. The patient brought a sinus CT scan with him performed 3 months earlier that demonstrated pansinusitis with air-fluid levels in the frontal, maxillary, and sphenoid sinuses.

Based on the above history and examination, the patient was offered the option of revision endoscopic sinus surgery to which he consented.

HEADLINE NEWS

After initial evaluation and discussion of surgery with the patient, the senior author was approached by a national television news show interested in producing a segment on sinusitis, highlighting its newest treatment options. The patient was asked if he would be willing to be interviewed for a news segment and have portions of his surgery televised on a national show. The patient expressed interest and was subsequently interviewed on camera with the senior author. An endoscopic sinus surgery with image guidance was performed, and a filming crew was present during portions of the surgery, which was later broadcast on national news.

The performance of operations in front of live audiences has had its place in the surgical theater for hundreds of years. Surgeons used to routinely perform procedures in an amphitheater setting with interested students, trainees, and members of the general public in attendance.[1,2] The value of observation and dissemination of knowledge to larger groups of learners has been argued in the literature.[2–4] It has been suggested that the broadcast of live surgeries can spread firsthand experience of uncommon procedures to a larger group of trainees,[3] and that it can improve the informed consent process by providing firsthand experience to the public.[2]

On the other hand, the performance of surgery with a broadcast crew present in the operating room raises certain ethical issues that need to be considered. Some authors have noted that selection of the surgeon is important, and that they must not "be swept by the fever of the live setting," suggesting that not all surgeons are capable of handling the scenario, although the authors do not mention how the selection should be made.[3] Additionally, it has been suggested that live surgery may lead to increased time pressures,[2] decreased success rates,[5,6] and a hesitation to abort the novel procedure even with the risk of a poor clinical outcome.[2,4,7] A prime example of this was a well-publicized death after a live surgery in 2015. The primary surgeon was demonstrating a laparoscopic liver resection technique during a live broadcast and ran into heavy bleeding. The surgeon did not abandon his approach for several hours, and ultimately the patient died in the intensive care unit after surgery, emphasizing the inherent conflict of interest between the surgeon demonstrating a new technique for an audience and the patient undergoing the procedure.[8]

Despite the ethical debate, live demonstrations and broadcasts are here to stay, and will likely represent an increasing part of medicine and medical education in the future. The operating surgeon has the responsibility to balance the benefits and risks of broadcasted surgery, and ensure that the patient is adequately informed to participate in the decision process.

TREATMENT

The initial televised endoscopic surgery was performed without complication. The patient underwent bilateral sphenoethoidectomy with frontal sinus drill out (also known as a Draf 3 or Modified Lothrop Procedure). Two years later, the patient presented with recurrent sinonasal symptoms, despite ongoing medical therapy. Repeat computed tomography (CT) scan demonstrated re-opacification for the frontal sinuses, and he underwent revision frontal sinus drillout, again without complication. Despite initial symptomatic relief, his infections recurred and progressively worsened over the next 3 years. He suffered from debilitating frontal headaches requiring repeated courses of antibiotics. Endoscopic examination demonstrated restenosis of the frontal sinus drillout site, and CT scan showed persistent frontal sinus opacification. Five years after his intial drillout procedure, the patient underwent osteoplastic flap obliteration of the frontal sinuses.

Frontal sinus obliteration was performed via brow incision with elevation of an osteoplastic flap. The infected sinuses were thoroughly cleaned of infected mucosa and obliterated with abdominal fat. The case went well, but the patient had significant bucking and hypertension on emergence from anesthesia. Shortly after arriving in the recovery room, he complained of left eye pain. Examination revealed a tense, proptotic left eye with an unreactive pupil and no light perception. An immediate lateral canthotomy and cantholysis was performed at the bedside under local anesthesia (Figure 15–1). Prompt ophthalmologic consultation was obtained, and the patient was administered IV dexamethasone and acetazolamide. He was returned to the operating room where he underwent left endoscopic medial orbital decompression with removal of the entire lamina papyracea and incision of the underlying periorbita to reduce intraorbital pressure. The ophthalmologist performed a superior orbital exploration. Upon return to the recovery room, the patient was able to count fingers with his left eye at 3 feet. The patient was admitted after surgery, and his visual acuity returned to baseline after surgery.

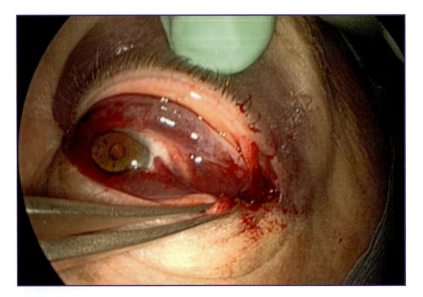

Figure 15–1. Left orbital hematoma after the performance of sinus surgery. A lateral canthotomy and cantholysis have been performed to reduce intraorbital and intraocular pressures.

FOLLOW-UP

At his first follow-up visit 1 week after surgery, the patient was noted to have some periorbital ecchymosis, and the canthotomy incision, which had intentionally not been sutured closed, was healing well (Figure 15–2). Three months after surgery, his visual acuity on ophthalmologic exam matched that of his preoperative level (Figure 15–3). In addition, his preoperative frontal headaches had resolved and did not return in the next 3 years of follow-up.

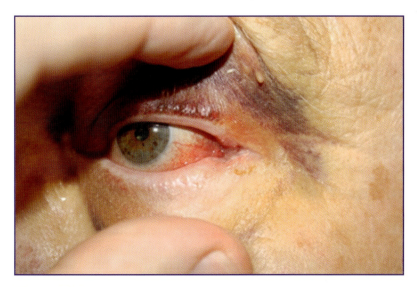

Figure 15–2. One-week postoperative visit. Residual periorbital ecchymosis with satisfactory healing of the lateral canthal incision are noted.

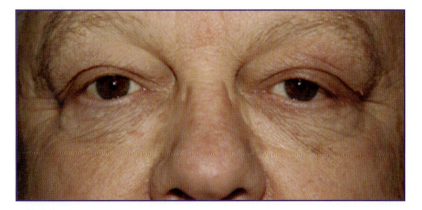

Figure 15–3. Three-month postoperative visit. Patient's ophthalmological examination, including visual acuity, is normal.

MANAGEMENT OF ORBITAL HEMATOMA

The management in this case was fortunate because the complication was recognized early, and the patient did not have any long-term sequelae. Multiple authors acknowledge the importance of prompt action once an orbital hematoma is suspected. After recognition, nasal packing should be removed, lateral canthotomy preformed to reduce intraorbital pressure, and ophthalmologic consultation obtained.[9-11] Medical therapy should be initiated immediately, consisting of IV dexamethasone (8–10 mg IV every 8 hours for 3–4 doses) or IV mannitol (1–2 g/kg over 30 mintues), in order to decrease the intraocular pressure,[11] as well as the addition of acetazolamide to decrease the production of aqueous humor. Surgical therapy should be considered with visual compromise or worsening symptoms. Lateral canthotomy and cantholysis should be first line, with consideration of subsequent endoscopic orbital decompression as these maneuvers will contribute to a decrease in intraocular pressure and help preserve perfusion of the globe.[9-11]

THIS CASE WAS SCARY BECAUSE

The patient presented with an unexpected complication resulting in a return to the operating room, risk of loss of blindness, and prolongation of his hospital stay. Inevitably, discussion of disclosure arises when faced with a complication during a surgical case, and how best to approach the discussion with the family. Previous papers support the idea that disclosure is ethically obligatory due to the principles of respect and autonomy,[12-15] and that patients respond favorably to physician disclosure and explanation of the adverse event.[16,17] Indeed it seems that patients want to know about all errors involved in their care and may be more likely to forego punitive reimbursement if they feel that their physician has been attentive and honest.[17]

Complicating the care of this patient was his role as the subject of a national news story and high-profile, "very important" patient (VIP). Several reports have been published on the care of the high-profile or special patient, noting that care is often complicated by the patient's public or professional status. These authors mention that patients often come to harm because normal administrative and clinical routines are bypassed in order to provide a different level of care because of the patient's status.[18-20] Several principles are expounded upon in these papers, resisting involving senior physicians who normally would not be involved,[18,19] ensuring privacy and professionalism,[18-20] and that the physician should not withdraw from the patient due to the severity of illness.[20] In addition, the physician faces his or her own desire to provide paramount care to the VIP, as this may result in increased name recognition for the physician, more referrals, or expansion of his or her practice (Table 15–1).

The scenario presented in this chapter describes a major, vision-threatening complication of sinus surgery. It elucidates the immediate steps taken to reduce the likelihood of long-term morbidity. Fortunately, this patient involved had a favorable outcome. Although such a complication is a well-recognized risk of sinus surgery, the question remains as to whether or not the "high-profile" status of this patient influenced the management and care of this "scary case."

Table 15–1. Issues with Care of High-Profile Patients (public exposure, change your usual routine, desire to please, fear of complication/hope for more referrals, overtreatment)

Issues in the Care of the VIP Patient	
Benefits	**Obstacles**
Recognition	"Chairperson's syndrome"
Referrals	Alteration of routine and treatment
Expansion of practice	Protection of privacy
	Prevention of withdrawal from patient

REFERENCES

1. Williams JB, Mathews R, D'Amico TA. "Reality surgery"—a research ethics perspective on the live broadcast of surgical procedures. *J Surg Educ.* 2011 Jan-Feb;68(1):58–61. doi: 10.1016/j.jsurg.2010.08.009. Epub 2010 Nov 5. Review.
2. Essex-Lopresti M. Operating theatre design. *Lancet.* 1999;353:1007–1010.
3. Vanermen H. Live surgery should not be outlawed at national and regional cardiothoracic meetings. *J Thorac Cardiovasc Surg.* 2010;4:822–825.
4. Kallmes DF, Cloft HJ, Molyneux A, Burger I, Brinjikji W, Murphy KP. Live case demonstrations: patient safety, ethics, consent, and conflicts. *Lancet.* 2011 Apr 30;377(9776):1539–1541. doi: 10.1016/S0140-6736(11)60357-7.
5. Chatelain P, Meier B, de la Serna F, et al. Success with coronary angioplasty as seen at demonstrations of procedure. *Lancet.* 1992 Nov 14;340(8829):1202–1205.
6. Liao Z, Li ZS, Leung JW, et al. How safe and successful are live demonstrations of therapeutic ERCP? A large multicenter study. *Am J Gastroenterol,.*2009;104:47–52.
7. Franke J, Reimers B, Scarpa M, et al. Complications of carotid stenting during live transmissions. *JACC Cardiovasc Interv.* 2009 Sep;2(9):887–891.
8. Nagarajan R. Patient dies during live demo surgery at AIIMS, sparks ethics row. *The Times of India.* http://news.doximity.com/entries/1898706?user_id=211432
9. Patel AB, Hoxworth JM, Lal D. Orbital complications associated with the treatment of chronic rhinosinusitis. *Otolaryngol Clin North Am.* 2015 Jun 24. 48(5):749–768.
10. Bhatti MT, Stankiewicz JA. Ophthalmic complications of endoscopic sinus surgery. *Surv Ophthalmol.* 2003;48(4):389–402.
11. Ramakrishnan VR, Palmer JN. Prevention and management of orbital hematoma. *Otolaryngol Clin North Am.* 2010;43(4):789–800.
12. Bluebond-Langner R, Rodriguez ED, Wu AW. Discussing adverse outcomes with patients and families. *Oral Maxillofac Surg Clin North Am.* 2010 Nov;22(4):471–479.
13. Mazor KM, Simon SR, Yood RA, et al. Health plan members' views about disclosure of medical errors. *Ann Intern Med.* 2004;140(6):409–418, E419–423.
14. Bluebond-Langner R, Rodriguez ED, Wu AW. Discussing adverse outcomes with patients and families. *Oral Maxillofac Surg Clin North Am.* 2010 Nov;22(4):471–479.
15. Lipira LE, Gallagher TH. Disclosure of adverse events and errors in surgical care: challenges and strategies for improvement. *World J Surg.* 2014 Jul;38(7):1614–1621.

16. Mazor KM, Simon SR, Yood RA, et al. Health plan members' views on forgiving medical errors. *Am J Manag Care*. 2005 Jan;11(1):49–52.
17. Witman AB, Park DM, Hardin SB. How do patients want physicians to handle mistakes? A survey of internal medicine patients in an academic setting. *Arch Intern Med*. 1996 Dec 9-23;156(22):2565–2569.
18. Smith MS, Shesser RF. The emergency care of the VIP patient. *N Engl J Med*. 1988;319:1421–1423.
19. Guzman JA, Sasidhar M, Stoller JK. Caring for VIPs: nine principles. *Cleve Clin J Med*. 2011 Feb;78(2):90–94.
20. Schneck SA. "Doctoring" doctors and their families. *JAMA*. 1998 Dec 16;280(23):2039–2042.

CHAPTER 16

Facial Nerve Injury

The Service Recovery Paradox

Kimberly A. Russell
Robert W. Dolan

THE CASE

A 56-year-old woman was referred to a tertiary care center for treatment of a parotid tumor. Her problems began with headaches for which a magnetic resonance imaging (MRI) scan of her head was obtained. The MRI scan did not find a cause for her headaches but another incidental lesion was seen. She was found to have a deep lobe of parotid mass that was not felt to have any relationship to her headaches (Figure 16–1). The mass was asymptomatic and the initial 2 otolaryngologists whom she had seen could not palpate the mass. Because the mass was not palpable, the initial treating otolaryngologist sent her for a core needle biopsy with an interventional radiologist.

The interventional radiologist performed an image-guided needle biopsy under local anesthesia. In an effort to obtain sufficient tissue for diagnosis, a large-gauge needle was inserted into the mass for sampling. The patient immediately experienced a sharp pain, followed by a complete ipsilateral facial paralysis. This was an unexpected complication, but even more concerning was the pathology report from the biopsy that was "suspicious for malignancy."

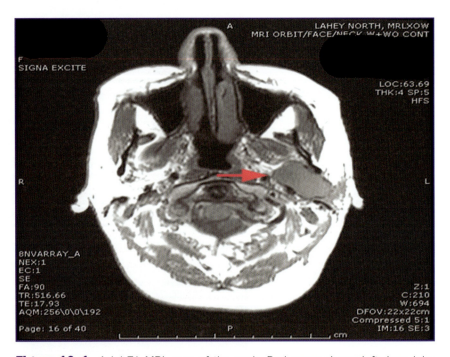

Figure 16–1. Axial T1 MRI scan of the neck. Red arrow shows left deep lobe parotid mass.

The patient was distressed, having encountered a complete facial paresis from this procedure and a potential malignant diagnosis (Figure 16–2). She sought the opinion of another otolaryngologist who planned for a standard approach parotidectomy. She underwent surgical exploration of a left deep lobe of parotid mass. During the procedure, the facial nerve was found to be superficial and splayed over the mass and would not electrically stimulate. The mass was deemed "unresectable," and she was referred to our tertiary medical center for definitive care of this parotid tumor and her complete facial paresis, which did not improve following core needle biopsy.

During our initial evaluation, she was clearly distraught, with disfigurement from the complete facial nerve paralysis resulting in difficulty speaking and eating. She also thought she had cancer based on the needle biopsy. Finally, she had prior experiences with medical care that did not meet her expectations. We discussed the need for a definitive diagnosis and removal of the mass that appeared resectable on subsequent imaging.

She subsequently underwent a transcervical approach to the infratemporal fossa. Surgery included translocation of the submandibular gland, transection of the stylomandibular

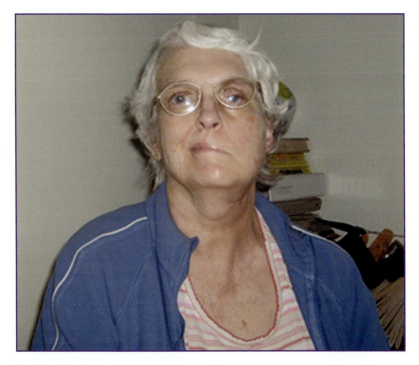

Figure 16–2. Left facial nerve paresis.

and omohyoid ligaments, division of the external carotid artery, excision of the deep lobe parotid tumor, and neurorrhaphy of the facial nerve. She had an uneventful postoperative recovery. Postoperatively, she was seen in our office every 2 weeks until her facial movement began to recover (Figure 16–3). Final pathology revealed benign pleomorphic adenoma. She regained movement in her face within several months with a final House-Brackmann score of II. Despite her ordeal and residual facial paralysis, she stated that she was extremely grateful and appreciative of the care she received (Figure 16–4)!

THIS CASE WAS SCARY BECAUSE

Whenever a patient has sought multiple opinions, there is increased risk due to either a complex problem, or a challenging patient. We were her third opinion for a mass in a difficult location. A potential diagnosis for a malignant tumor is scary.

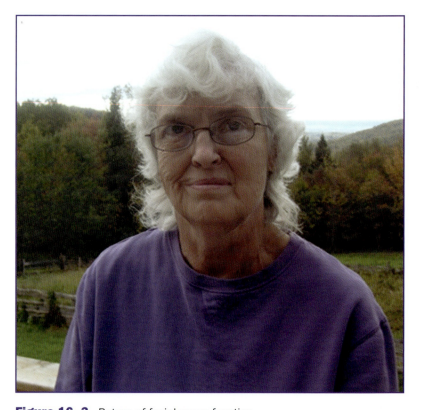

Figure 16–3. Return of facial nerve function.

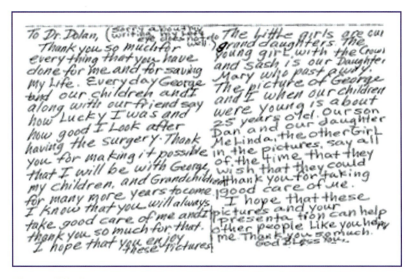

Figure 16–4. Letter of gratitude from the patient to Dr. Dolan.

The patient already had a very bad outcome at the time of her initial evaluation by our clinic. She already had a major complication with a total left-sided facial paralysis. The possibility of future litigation was present as well as her mistrust with the medical profession. She started with an asymptomatic, incidental finding that turned out benign, yet she is left with a residual facial deficit.

WHAT I LEARNED FROM THIS CASE

First, core needle biopsies of the parotid gland can cause serious injury and should be used in very select cases where fine needle or open resection cannot be performed. There are differing opinions regarding the use of needle biopsy for parotid lesions, but the risk of core needle biopsy is much greater than fine needle within the parotid glands.

This case demonstrated an example of *The Service Recovery Paradox*. The Service Recovery Paradox states, with a highly effective service recovery, a service or product failure is transformed into an experience that surpasses the satisfaction ratings from "customers" more than if the failure had never happened. This is a concept that applies to this case. The patient experienced a very turbulent treatment course with an initial diagnosis that was wrong, posttreatment permanent partial facial nerve paralysis, and invasive diagnostic procedures all for what was ultimately determined to be a benign tumor. Nevertheless, she became extremely satisfied with her care and her satisfaction was much more than what is typically experienced for a patient with an uneventful treatment course. The clinician should be aware of the remarkable phenomenon of extreme satisfaction with care that is possible despite an objectively poor initial experience and poorer than typical final outcome.

We should all strive for the Service Recovery Paradox when dealing with major complications. When a complication is encountered, the natural inclination is to want to avoid seeing that patient and having to deal with the event. For a surgeon to experience a major complication, every time he or she sees the patient, he or she is reminded of the error, the grief, and the potential liability that is involved. These visits also usually take more time to answer questions and explain prognoses to patients. However, patients who experience complications need to be seen more often than usual to achieve the Service Recovery Paradox. Clinicians often make themselves available to patients and families with personal contacts and daily inpatient visits when a complication has occurred.

LEGAL COMMENTARY: Anthony Abeln, JD

When dealing with complications of another physician, it is important to communicate honestly with the patient and the referring providers. The number one reason cited in studies for medical malpractice claims is a negative comment by another physician. It is easier for the second opinion to have 100% hindsight into the correct actions, but he or she was not present for the initial treatment and there were usually circumstances that they were unaware of that contributed to the complication. It is often best to reserve judgments and opinions until all the facts are known and focus on providing the best care to ensure recovery of the patients.

CHAPTER 17

Encephalocele

An Unexpected Finding

Jonathon Sillman

THE CASE

A 53-year-old patient presented with left ear pain and drainage, intermittent for many years. He had a mild hearing loss as well, but denied any dizziness, imbalance, or headaches. He had a lifelong history of eustachian tube dysfunction and had myringotomy with tubes as a child. He was treated by another otolaryngologist with oral and topical antibiotics with temporary improvement of his ear symptoms. His past history was significant for a kidney transplant with immunosuppressive medications.

On his initial presentation, examination showed normal pinnae bilaterally. The right ear canal was normal, and the right tympanic membrane showed mild retraction. On the left side the ear canal was normal, but the tympanic membrane was diffusely edematous and erythematous, with no perforation. The nasopharynx was normal as was the rest of the nose and throat exam. He was treated with Augmentin and Ciprodex drops and returned with examination showing a clear but retracted left tympanic membrane onto a partially eroded incus. There was no perforation, granulation tissue, or squamous debris. The right ear exam was unchanged. Audiometry showed a mild bilateral conductive hearing loss.

The patient did well for 3 months, but then developed recurrent left otorrhea. Exam showed granulation tissue within a left tympanic membrane retraction pocket, again with no perforation or squamous debris. The otorrhea improved with Ciprodex, but the patient continued to have granulation tissue in the left tympanic membrane retraction pocket. A left tympanoplasty was recommended to correct the retraction pocket and prevent further ossicular erosion.

THE SURGERY

At the time of surgery, which was performed with the assistance of a resident in an ambulatory surgical center, granulation tissue was found to be extending onto the posterior ear canal wall from the retraction pocket (Figure 17–1). The initial procedure was carried out using a 0-degree endoscope. A decision was made to resect the posterior canal skin encompassing the granulation tissue, and this was sent for permanent pathology to rule out malignancy. Following this excision, a tympanomeatal flap was elevated and the middle ear was entered. The middle ear was found to have mild to moderate mucosal edema, some mucoid fluid, but no evidence of cholesteatoma. The incus

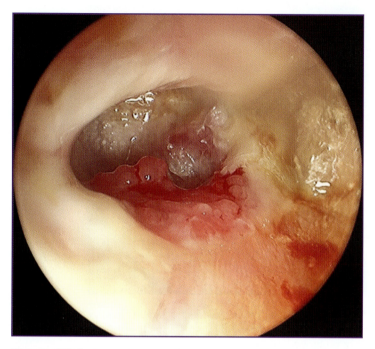

Figure 17–1. Operative view of the ear canal. There is granulation tissue extending onto the posterior ear canal wall from the retraction pocket.

long process was found to be eroded, but the stapes was intact and mobile (Figure 17–2). An attempt was made to repair the incus erosion with hydroxyapatite cement (Figure 17–3); however, the cement cracked on placing a fascia graft under the tympanic membrane remnant, and a decision was made to perform ossicular reconstruction using either an incus interposition graft or using a titanium partial ossicular replacement prosthesis (PORP). Upon separating the incus from the malleus head with an attic hook, the incus came out smoothly followed by copious clear fluid!

THE UNEXPECTED

The resident remarked that perhaps this was "run down of local anesthetic"; however, the attending immediately knew better: this was cerebrospinal fluid. A postauricular approach was then performed under the microscope, and an atticotomy was performed revealing a significant tegmen encephalocele (Figure 17–4) surrounding the malleus head. The encephalocele was mobilized off the malleus and the malleus head was resected (Figure 17–5).

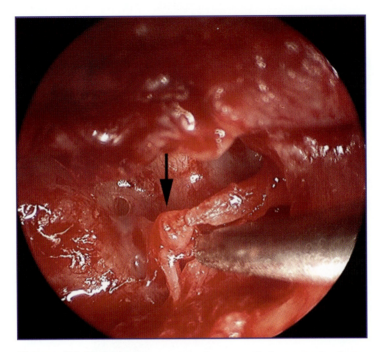

Figure 17–2. Middle ear exploration revealed mucosal edema, mucoid fluid, but no evidence of cholesteatoma. The incus long process was found to be eroded, but the stapes (*arrow*) was intact and mobile.

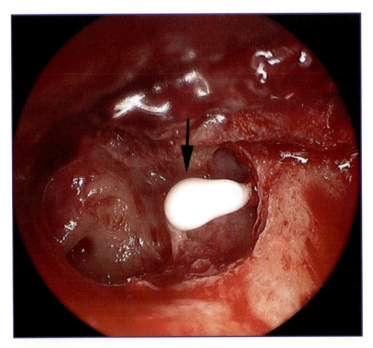

Figure 17–3. An attempt was made to repair the incus erosion with hydroxyapatite cement (*arrow*).

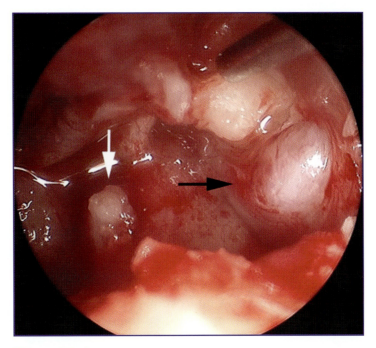

Figure 17–4. Upon removing the incus, an unexpected tegmen encephalocele (*black arrow*) was encountered (*white arrow* = stapes).

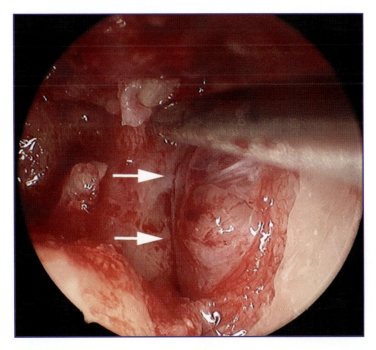

Figure 17–5. The encephalocele (*arrows*) was mobilized off the malleus and the malleus head was resected.

The encephalocele was then reduced with bipolar cautery (Figure 17–6A). The bony edges of the tegmen defect were defined, and a conchal cartilage graft was placed into the space between dura and tegmen bone from below (Figure 17–6B). A layer of SurgiMend was then placed beneath the cartilage graft and tucked above the tegmen bone edges (Figure 17–6C).

A titanium PORP with cartilage graft was then placed, the epitympanum and mesotympanum were packed with collagen sponge, and the remaining tympanomeatal flap was laid over the posterior canal wall. The ear canal was packed with collagen sponge and Otopore sponge and the postauricular wound was closed in the usual fashion, followed by a mastoid dressing. The patient was transferred for admission to the hospital for observation. A neurosurgery colleague was consulted. The patient underwent computed tomography (CT) (Figure 17–7)

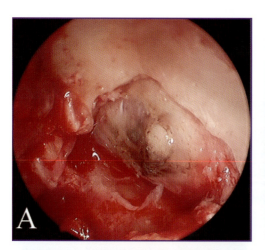
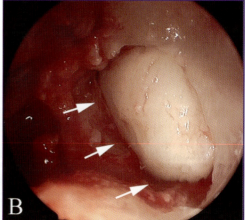
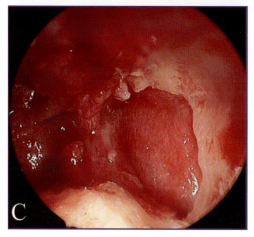

Figure 17–6. **A.** The encephalocele was then reduced with bipolar cautery. **B.** The bony edges of the tegmen defect were defined, and a conchal cartilage graft was placed into the space between dura and tegmen bone from below. **C.** A layer of SurgiMend was then placed beneath the cartilage graft and tucked above the tegmen bone edges.

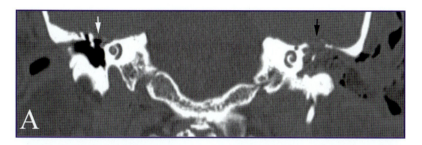
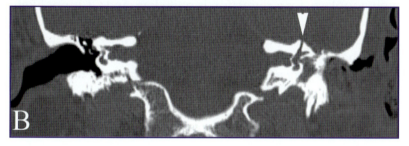

Figure 17–7. A. Postoperative CT scan of the temporal bones showed a right middle ear encephalocele (*white arrow*), left ear s/p encephalocele repair (*black arrow*). **B.** There were incidental bilateral superior semicircular canal dehiscences (*arrowhead*) that were not symptomatic and not repaired.

and magnetic resonance imaging (MRI) that showed no intracranial hemorrhage. The patient was observed overnight, had no neurologic sequelae, and was discharged home in good condition. He subsequently healed well, had a good hearing outcome, and has had no more otorrhea. Of note, his CT scan showed bilateral tegmen dehiscence and bilateral superior semicircular canal dehiscence, although he had no dizziness.

THIS CASE WAS SCARY BECAUSE

This case was scary because we were facing an unexpected, potentially dangerous intraoperative finding in an ambulatory surgical center, which was not equipped with the usual instrumentation one would want available to repair a temporal bone encephalocele. Craniotomy instruments, middle fossa retractor, and neurosurgical colleagues were not available. One could have decided to close the wound, transfer to the hospital, and complete repair in that setting; however, the tegmen defect was accessible and relatively limited such that a repair from below was deemed feasible. Being able to repair the defect at the time of the tympanoplasty saved the patient from a second anesthesia.

WHAT I LEARNED FROM THIS CASE

What I learned from the case is to expect the unexpected. I certainly have debated whether I should obtain preoperative CT scans on patients with tympanic membrane retractions, and in this case it would have led me to plan a procedure in the hospital in collaboration with neurosurgery. However, the likelihood of finding a tegmen encephalocele at the time of tympanoplasty for a retraction is quite low, and CT is not likely to be cost effective. I also learned that it is always worthwhile to clarify the unexpected situation as much as possible, take a step back, and allow yourself to make a reasoned decision as to how to proceed when the unexpected is encountered.

CASE OUTCOME

The patient has done well with good hearing (Figure 17–8) and resolution of his ear drainage. He was fully informed of the findings and was pleased with the outcome.

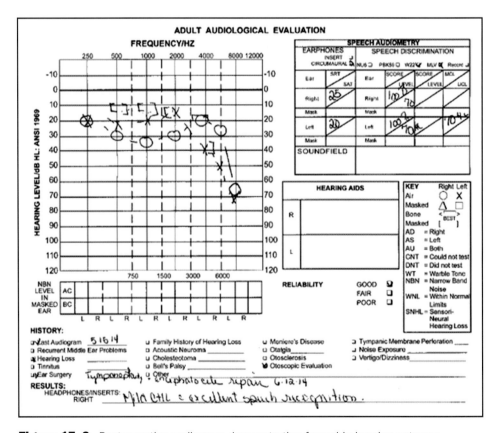

Figure 17–8. Postoperative audiogram demonstrating favorable hearing outcome.

# CHAPTER 18

Intracranial Extension

A Benign Disease?

Scharukh Jalisi
Avner Aliphas
Samuel J. Rubin
Kenneth M. Grundfast

THE CASE

A 31-year-old female with a history of congenital cholesteatoma who had several ear operations during childhood and then a canal wall down mastoidectomy at age 16 years was being followed with periodic routine mastoid cavity débridement every 6 months. At age 31, she mentioned during one of the routine mastoid débridements that she had transient right facial twitching that lasted for a few days and then resolved. There mastoid bowl was well epithelized, dry, with no sign of cholesteatoma. She was told to return in 6 months. At the next office visit for mastoid débridement, she said that the right-side facial twitching occurred again but resolved within a few days. In addition, she said that she was having headaches. She had been diagnosed with migraine headaches with ophthalmic auras. Medications consisted of amitriptyline and intermittent use of meclizine for dizziness. She worked as a business analyst at an investment firm and did not consume alcohol, smoke cigarettes, or use recreational drugs. She did not have a family history of otologic disease. On review of systems she did not have any new otologic complaints. Her dizziness did not interfere with her daily life, and she denied recent otorrhea or tinnitus.

There were no abnormal findings on the neurological exam with normal cranial nerve function, including cranial nerve VII. The otologic exam demonstrated a normal left ear while the microscopic exam of the right ear revealed a canal wall down cavity, a narrow meatus, and no cholesteatoma. A nasal endoscopy was performed without evidence of a nasopharyngeal mass. An audiogram was unchanged compared to prior audiograms and showed right-sided severe conductive hearing loss without a sensorineural hearing loss component (Figure 18–1). She had a speech reception threshold of 60 dB and a speech discrimination score of 100%.

Even though there were no unusual findings on examination of the right mastoid cavity, because of the recurring episodes of right facial twitching and transient right facial weakness, a computed tomography (CT) scan of the temporal bone was ordered. Surprisingly, the CT scan showed a right-sided soft tissue mass extending through the epitympanum into the middle cranial fossa. A more posterior view revealed a clear mastoid bowl with an intact tegmen on the right side (Figure 18–2). Subsequently, a T1-weighted post-gadolinium magnetic resonance imaging (MRI) scan revealed a nonenhancing iso-intense mass in the middle cranial fossa,

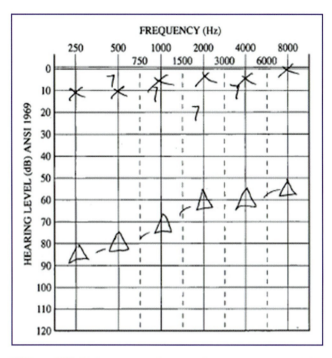

Figure 18–1. Patient audiogram describing severe right-sided conductive hearing loss without a sensorineural hearing loss component.

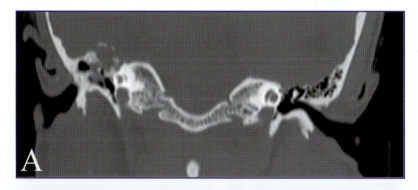
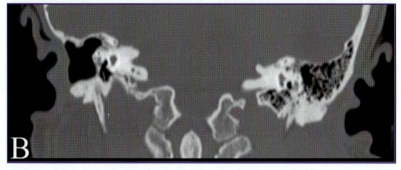

Figure 18–2. Preoperative CT scan of the temporal bones. Note that there is an expansile intracranial mass over the tegmen (**A**), despite having healthy and aerated mastoid cavity (**B**).

indicating a likely extradural mass, while a T2-weighted image revealed a hyperintense mass, increasing suspicion for a cholesteatoma (Figure 18–3).

THIS CASE WAS SCARY BECAUSE

This case was scary because for more than 15 years the mastoid bowl was periodically examined and débrided twice yearly, and there was no evidence of persistent or recurrent cholesteatoma on ear examination, but during much of this time the patient had an unrecognized enlarging intracranial middle fossa cholesteatoma mass that could have killed her. The cholesteatoma presumably had originated in tegmen air cells that were covered by epithelium giving the mastoid bowl a most ordinary appearance.

WHAT I LEARNED FROM THIS CASE

What I learned from this case is that cholesteatoma that remains in a tegmen air cell can develop into a mass that grows cephalad into the middle fossa and is not at all evident on examination of the ear in a canal wall down mastoid cavity. Management of congenital cholesteatoma is treacherous because the keratin growth usually occurs within a well-

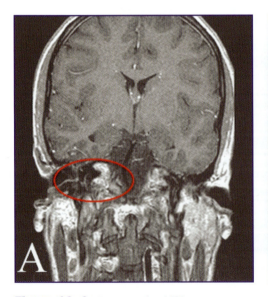 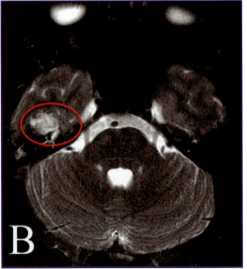

Figure 18–3. Preoperative MRI scan.

aerated mastoid with numerous air cell interstices so that complete removal of cholesteatoma is difficult and chances for recidivistic cholesteatoma are high. Whenever a patient with history of cholesteatoma develops facial twitching and/or transient facial weakness ipsilateral to the ear with cholesteatoma, then the patient should have a CT scan of temporal bones to look for middle fossa mass. In our case, the patient had a middle cranial fossa approach to resect the cholesteatoma mass (Figure 18–4). Quite likely, if this middle-age mother had not had the CT scan that revealed the middle fossa mass, she could have died from complications in management of a benign otologic condition that started in her childhood.

REVIEW OF LITERATURE

A cholesteatoma is a "non-neoplastic but destructive lesion containing layers of keratin in a cavity containing squamous epithelium and epithelial connective tissue."[1] While there are multiple theories regarding the formation of acquired cholesteatomas, the most likely explanation for the formation of congenital cholesteatomas is persistence of fetal epidermoid cells medial to the tympanic membrane.[1] Congenital cholesteatoma usually presents as spherical white cysts behind a normal tympanic membrane, and criteria for diagnosis include an intact tympanic membrane with no previous history of perforation

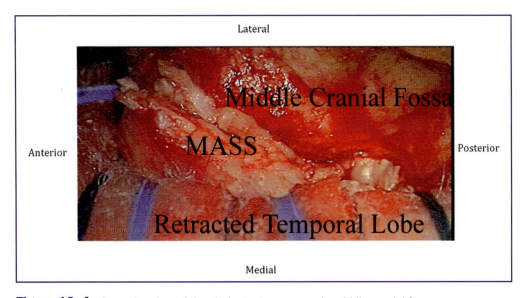

Figure 18–4. Operative view of the cholesteatoma mass in middle cranial fossa.

or otorrhea and no prior otologic surgery.[2,3] The annual incidence of cholesteatoma is 3 per 100,000 in children and 9.2 per 100,000 in adults with a male-to-female ratio of 1.4:1.[4] Furthermore, middle ear cholesteatoma is more common in people younger than 50 years of age.[4] Although cholesteatoma is a benign disease, it can lead to significant morbidity as a result of its destructive character.

It is often necessary to use preoperative imaging to determine the location of a cholesteatoma and possible destruction of surrounding structures. Barath et al. advocates the use of high-resolution CT for clinically suspected cholesteatoma because of its excellent spatial resolution, high sensitivity, and high negative predictive value.[4] However, CT has poor specificity, and it is difficult to differentiate between soft tissue structures such as granulation tissue, cholesterol granulomas, or neoplasm. Therefore, if there is suspicion that the mass is something other than a cholesteatoma, or if there is suspicion of intracranial invasion, magnetic resonance imaging should be used.[4]

The data are sparse when describing intracranial invasion of cholesteatoma, and there have not been any large-scale studies looking at prevalence, likely due to the rarity of this presentation. Nevertheless, there have been numerous case studies and case series on this topic.[5-13] Horn (2000) described one of the larger case series of intracranial invasion (both middle cranial fossa and posterior cranial fossa) including six subjects.[8] All six patients experienced hearing loss while 50% also experienced tinnitus. The most common presenting complaints included otorrhea, facial paralysis, and blepharospasm. Additionally, the most common passage for intracranial spread of the cholesteatoma was through the supratubal recess or anterior epitympanic air cell.

Two of the main surgical approaches for treatment of cholesteatoma include intact canal wall (ICW) mastoidectomy and canal wall down (CWD) mastoidectomy. The ICW mastoidectomy differs from the CWD mastoidectomy by preservation of the posterior wall of the external auditory canal. Some advantages of the ICW mastoidectomy include decreased aural care, more rapid healing, and allowance for water exposure (swimming).[14] While ICW mastoidectomy requires a 2-staged surgical procedure compared to the single-stage procedure used for CWD mastoidectomy, patients who receive ICW mastoidectomy demonstrate better postoperative hearing compared to the patients receiving the CWD mastoidectomy, and avoid creation of a large mastoid bowl.[15,16]

A meta-analysis conducted by Kerckhoffs et al determined that the recidivism rate was 0% to 13.2% for patients receiving CWD mastoidectomy compared to a recidivism rate of 16.7% to 61% in patients receiving ICW mastoidectomy.[17] However, the mean follow-up period in the studies included did not exceed 10 years. Waidyasekara et al and Sheehy et al both describe cases of cholesteatoma recurrence more than 20 years after modified radical mastoidectomy for the initial cholesteatoma, indicating that cholesteatomas can present many years after initial treatment.[6,11] Some of the predictive factors of residual cholesteatoma include posterior mesotympanum involvement, ossicular chain interruption after disease excision, primary surgery before the age of 8 years, or mastoid involvement.[18,19]

CASE OUTCOME

During postoperative follow-up, the patient's facial twitching resolved, but she continued to experience occasional migraines. A postoperative MRI showed no evidence of residual cholesteatoma (Figure 18–5). The patient has had no recurrence of cholesteatoma or neurologic deficits 10 years after the intracranial surgery.

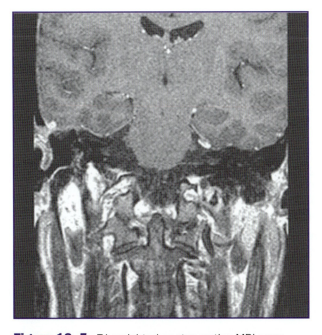

Figure 18–5. T1 weighted postoperative MRI scan.

REFERENCES

1. Persaud R, Hajioff D, Trinidade A, et al. Evidence-based review of aetiopathogenic theories of congenital and acquired cholesteatoma. *J Laryngol Otol.* 2007;121(11):1013–1019.
2. Isaacson G. Diagnosis of pediatric cholesteatoma. *Pediatrics.* 2007;120(3):603–608.
3. Levenson MJ, Parisier SC, Chute P, Wenig S, Juarbe C. A review of twenty congenital cholesteatomas of the middle ear in children. *Otolaryngol Head Neck Surg.* 1986;94(5):560–567.
4. Baráth K, Huber AM, Stämpfli P, Varga Z, Kollias S. Neuroradiology of cholesteatomas. *AJNR Am J Neuroradiol.* 2011;32(2):221–229.
5. Hanson JR, Esquivel C, Backous DD. Diagnosis and management of aggressive, acquired cholesteatoma with skull base and calvarial involvement: a report of 3 cases. *Am J Otolaryngol.* 2006;27(4):291–294.
6. Sheehy JL. Residual cholesteatoma in the middle cranial fossa. A case report. *Am J Otol.* 1984;5(3):227–228.
7. Rashad U, Hawthorne M, Kumar U, Welsh A. Unusual cases of congenital cholesteatoma of the ear. *J Laryngol Otol.* 1999;113(1):52–54.
8. Horn KL. Intracranial extension of acquired aural cholesteatoma. *Laryngoscope.* 2000;110(5 pt 1):761–772.
9. Rapoport PB, Di Francesco RC, Mion O, Bento RF. Huge congenital cholesteatoma simulating an intracranial abscess. *Otolaryngol Head Neck Surg.* 2000;123(1 pt 1):148–149.
10. Watanabe K, Hatano GY, Fukada N, Kawasaki T, Aoki H, Yagi T. Brain abscess secondary to the middle ear cholesteatoma: a report of two cases. *Auris Nasus Larynx.* 2004;31(4):433–437.
11. Waidyasekara P, Dowthwaite SA, Stephenson E, Bhuta S, Mcmonagle B. Massive temporal lobe cholesteatoma. *Case Rep Otolaryngol.* 2015;doi:10.1155/2015/121028.
12. Kreutzer EW, Deblanc GB. Extra-aural spread of acquired cholesteatoma. A report of two unique cases. *Arch Otolaryngol.* 1982;108(5):320–323.
13. Chu FW, Jackler RK. Anterior epitympanic cholesteatoma with facial paralysis: a characteristic growth pattern. *Laryngoscope.* 1988;98(3):274–279.
14. Schraff SA, Strasnick B. Pediatric cholesteatoma: a retrospective review. *Int J Pediatr Otorhinolaryngol.* 2006;70(3):385–393.
15. Osborn AJ, Papsin BC, James AL. Clinical indications for canal wall-down mastoidectomy in a pediatric population. *Otolaryngol Head Neck Surg.* 2012;147(2):316–322.
16. Grundfast KM, Ahuja GS, Parisier SC, Culver SM. Delayed diagnosis and fate of congenital cholesteatoma (keratoma). *Arch Otolaryngol Head Neck Surg.* 1995;121(8):903–907.
17. Kerckhoffs KG, Kommer MB, Van strien TH, et al. The disease recurrence rate after the canal wall up or canal wall down technique in adults. *Laryngoscope.* 2016;126(4):980–987.

18. Roger G, Denoyelle F, Chauvin P, Schlegel-stuhl N, Garabedian EN. Predictive risk factors of residual cholesteatoma in children: a study of 256 cases. *Am J Otol.* 1997;18(5):550–558.
19. Ahn SH, Oh SH, Chang SO, Kim CS. Prognostic factors of recidivism in pediatric cholesteatoma surgery. *Int J Pediatr Otorhinolaryngol.* 2003;67(12):1325–1330.

CHAPTER 19

Skull Base Injury

A Scary Harpoon

Ameer T. Shah
Walid I. Dagher

THE CASE

A 52-year-old male patient with a significant psychiatric history, and previous failed suicide attempts, called 911 after a repeat suicide attempt. He was unresponsive to the call operator. Emergency medical services arrived at his home and found the patient with a 3-foot-long metal rod with the entry point in the submental area and an exit point through the scalp (Figures 19–1 and 19–2). He was emergently fiberoptically orally

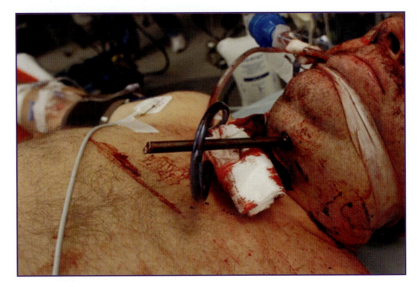

Figure 19–1. Entry point into submental area.

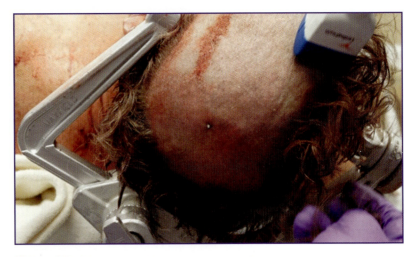

Figure 19–2. Exit point through parietal scalp area.

intubated on the scene and transferred to our facility for further management. The patient was noted to be hemodynamically stable upon presentation with a Glasgow Coma Scale of 3T. Due to the length of the metallic rod, he was unable to be placed within the computed tomography (CT) scanner gantry. After manual stabilization of the spear, the hospital maintenance team cut the metal rod to an appropriate length allowing entry into the CT scan gantry. A plain film x-ray was obtained to assess the extent of the injury. The metallic rod was consistent with a fishing spear with barb-like fins at its tip (Figure 19–3). A CT scan of the brain, cervical spine, and face were obtained revealing an entry point at the right submandibular region tracking through the skull base just lateral to the brainstem, with injury to the petrous portion of the left internal carotid artery (ICA), left frontal and temporal lobes and partial extrusion through the left temporoparietal bone (Figure 19–4). Due to the findings of carotid involvement, preoperative cerebral angiography was obtained, revealing adequate collateral circulation via the circle of Willis (Figure 19–5). The patient was then transferred to the operating room for surgical extraction of the foreign body.

Due to the vascular injury noted on imaging, it was deemed necessary to obtain proximal and distal vascular control. A combined team approach including Otolaryngology-Head and Neck Surgery and Neurosurgery was undertaken.

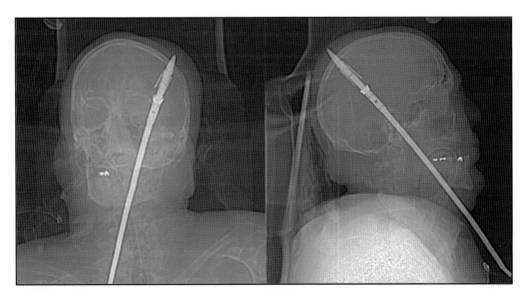

Figure 19–3. PA and lateral plain films showing the trajectory and characteristics of the penetrating object.

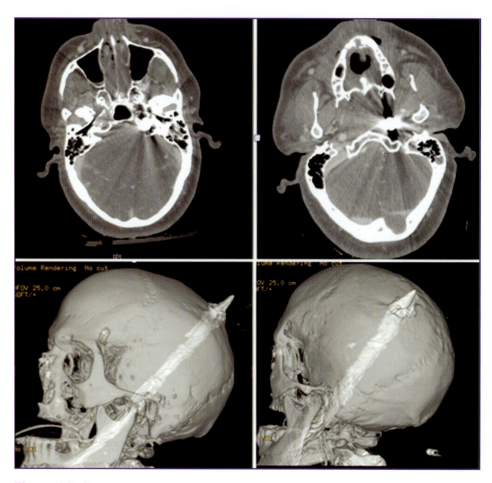

Figure 19–4. CT neck demonstrating in more detail the location and trajectory of the foreign body, specifically involvement of the petrous portions of the temporal bone and internal carotid artery. Lower images show 3D reformats.

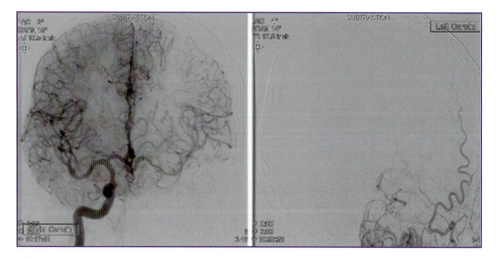

Figure 19–5. Coronal view of cerebral angiography demonstrates damage to the left internal carotid system.

The visible proximal edge of the spear was smoothed with a mastoid drill to minimize soft tissue injury upon forward extraction. A standard apron incision was designed and subplatysmal flaps were raised. The sternocleidomastoid muscles were lateralized allowing exposure of both carotid sheaths. The common, internal and external carotid arteries were isolated bilaterally. Vessel loops were placed around these arteries, securing proximal control. A skin flap was raised (Figure 19–6), and a left frontoparietal craniotomy was performed by the Neurosurgical team, exposing the dura and identifying the tip of the spear (Figure 19–7). The dura was

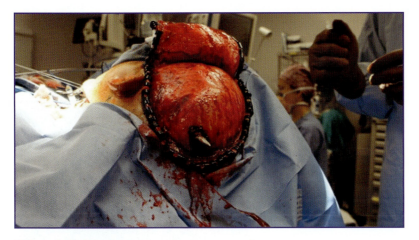

Figure 19–6. Skin flap raised prior to craniotomy exposing top of spear.

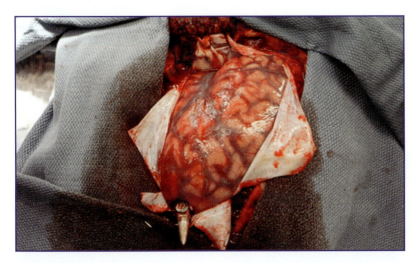

Figure 19–7. Left frontoparietal craniotomy and dura opened with exposure of Sylvian fissure.

then entered and the Sylvian fissure was identified. Access to the ICA was achieved by splitting the Sylvian fissure and following the olfactory and optic nerves until the ICA could be identified (Figure 19–8). Vessel loops were placed securing distal control. Once proximal and distal vascular control was secured, removal of the spear proceeded very slowly in an anterograde fashion, along the initial trajectory of the spear, to prevent deployment of the barbs. After successful removal (Figure 19–9), no bleeding was noted at the entry point in the neck, the oral cavity, or intracranially. The incisions were then closed and the patient was transferred intubated to the Neurosurgical ICU. Postoperatively the patient was continued on broad-spectrum antibiotics (ceftriaxone, vancomycin, and metronidazole) covering for oral flora. In addition, an Infectious Disease consultation was obtained to extend coverage to fresh water (*Aeromonas, Edwardsiella tarda*) and potential

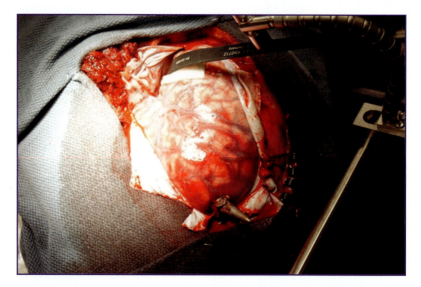

Figure 19–8. Retraction of Sylvian fissure to access circle of Willis.

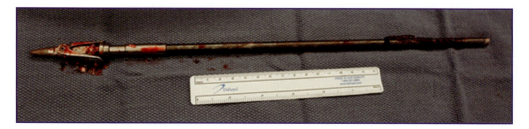

Figure 19–9. Spear after removal.

saltwater (*Vibrio vulnificus*) organisms. The patient remained intubated for several days postoperatively. Upon lightening his sedation, he was able to follow commands though was noted to have right-sided hemiplegia. He was successfully weaned off the ventilator and later extubated. A formal cerebral angiography revealed complete thrombosis of the left petrous carotid with no posttraumatic pseudoaneurysm formation and good collateral circle of Willis circulation. Eleven days after removal of the spear, the patient developed fevers despite broad antibiotic coverage. Magnetic resonance imaging of the brain revealed rim-enhancing fluid collections along the tract of the spear, raising suspicion for abscess formation. He was taken back to the operating room for exploration. No empyema was noted; however, there was evidence of brain parenchymal necrosis adjacent to the exit site, suggestive of cerebritis, though cultures were negative for organisms. The patient continued to show very slow improvement in his neurologic status and upon the family's interpretation of the patients' wishes, and after approval from the hospital ethics committee, the patient was designated do not resuscitate (DNR)/do not intubate (DNI). He was transferred to hospice and expired on day 33 following his suicide attempt.

This case was scary from the Otolaryngology standpoint for several reasons, including airway management, management of vascular injuries, and the infectious sequelae.

AIRWAY MANAGEMENT

This case is a perfect example to illustrate the management of a difficult airway. Although the intubation was done at the scene by a skilled EMS team, prior to the patient's presentation to our facility, few points about airway management are worth discussing. In any trauma patient, the neck is placed in a neutral position due to the high risk of cervical spine instability. A rapid sequence induction is usually performed as the PO status of these patients is unknown. Application of positive pressure ventilation achieves a high oxygen saturation, allowing an increased apnea time to secure the airway. Afterward, adequate visualization of the airway is imperative for successful intubation. Our case was challenging since many of these factors were not attainable. Because of the trauma sustained, the head-tilt chin lift method could not utilized. In addition, mouth opening was severely limited, prohibiting the placement of a laryngoscope. Application of face mask positive pressure ventilation was risky given the presence of an anterior skull base fracture. Although rare, face mask positive pressure ventilation has the potential to cause massive tension pneumocephalus with resultant increased intracranial pressure and eventually tonsillar herniation. Review of the literature identified only a few such cases of traumatic tension pneumocephalus after blunt head trauma and positive pressure ventilation. The literature, however, is abundant with reports of pneumocephalus after positive pressure ventilation in post skull base surgery patients.[1]

Additionally, concern has been expressed regarding the use of nasotracheal intubation in patients with facial fractures. Traditionally, the presence of facial trauma, particularly when it involves the bony structures of the midface and skull base, has been a contraindication for nasal intubation.[2] Although intracranial nasogastric tube placement in the presence of an anterior skull base fracture has been reported in the literature, only two cases of intracranial placement of nasotracheal tubes have been reported in association of an anterior skull base fracture.[3,4] Goodisson et al suggested that only the central anterior base of a skull fracture poses any risk of inadvertent intracranial nasotracheal tube placement and that fractures lying laterally and posteriorly do not pose such a problem. In cases where an anterior central base of skull fracture exists, fiberoptically assisted nasotracheal intubation allows safe passage of the endoscope through the nasopharynx and cords forming a stent along which an endotracheal tube can be passed safely.[5] In our patient, a fiberoptic nasotracheal intubation could not be achieved due to the trajectory of the spear into the nasopharynx narrowing it considerably and making navigation around it impossible. In the event of failed fiberoptic oral intubation, an awake tracheostomy would have been the alternative method to establish a secure airway. The presence of an experienced EMS team comfortable with difficult intubations played an important role in securing the airway.

VASCULAR INJURY

Another scary aspect to discuss is the technique for removal of the penetrating objects to the head and neck. Knowledge of the vascular anatomy of the head and neck area is paramount to the safe removal of penetrating foreign bodies. This case demonstrates the need to understand the vascular anatomy of the base of skull and the circle of Willis, as the management revolved around obtaining proximal and distal vascular control prior to removal of the foreign body. The literature is generally inconsistent in recommendations regarding blind removal vs removal under direct visualization. Some studies support blind removal; however, blind removal can be associated with an unacceptably high risk of further injury and death. High-resolution CT scan, plus CT angiogram or cerebral angiography, are critical in evaluating the soft tissue and brain parenchyma as well as how the foreign body relates to the surrounding vasculature. This allows for a higher success rate in avoiding vascular injury during removal.[6] With proximal and distal control of the vessels, the risk of vascular injury is minimized. The most common vascular sequelae include traumatic pseudoaneurysm, arteriovenous fistula, specifically carotid-cavernous fistula, subarachnoid hemorrhage, and vasospasm.[7] With respect to aneurysms, true aneurysms are uncommon, comprising less than 1%, with false pseudoaneurysms much more common, seen in up to 42% of patients.[8] These aneurysms may be delayed and have a 50% mortality rate if untreated.[9]

Last, infectious complications, such as meningitis, ventriculitis, cerebritis, and brain abscesses have been found in 48% to 64% of cases, with up to 20% of cases demonstrating sterile cultures, as seen in our patient.[6] It comes as no surprise that these confer a higher morbidity and mortality, and one should consider retained foreign body, bone fragments, skin, and hair along the tract. Factors associated with infectious sequelae include cerebrospinal fluid (CSF) leak, paranasal sinus involvement, transventricular injury, and wounds crossing the midline. Therefore along with considering return to the operating room for débridement and drainage, pharmacologic seizure prophylaxis and broad-spectrum antibiotics are indicated. *Staphylococcus aureus* is the most frequent causative organism; however, gram-negative bacteria are often implicated. In penetrating brain injury, ceftriaxone, metronidazole, and vancomycin is the recommended regimen, as was done in our patient. This is often continued for a period of 7 to 14 days.[7] One special consideration to make is the nature of the foreign body and whether additional antibiotics coverage is indicated. In our case, given that this was a harpoon injury, prophylactic coverage for specific marine flora was needed; therefore, consultation with Infectious Disease was a valuable resource.

WHAT I LEARNED FROM THIS CASE

This case demonstrates the intimate interaction between various specialties, and the importance of airway management and knowledge of the vascular anatomy of the head and neck. The increased utilization and availability of fiberoptic scopes for airway management has made cases like this more manageable; however, one should always be prepared for urgent or emergent tracheostomy when this is not available or possible. Though the morbidity and mortality are quite high with head and neck penetrating trauma extending intracranially, further injury and sequelae can be prevented through careful knowledge of the anatomy, planning, preoperative imaging when medically feasible, and cooperation via an interdisciplinary team approach.

REFERENCES

1. Nicholson B, Dhindsa H. Traumatic tension pneumocephalus after blunt head trauma and positive pressure ventilation. *Prehosp Emerg Care*. 2010 Oct–Dec; 14(4):499–504.
2. Marlow TJ, Goltra DD, Schabel SI. Intracranial placement of a nasotracheal tube after facial fracture: a rare complication. *J Emerg Med*. 1997 Mar–Apr; 15(2):187–191.
3. Horellou MF. Mathe D, Feiss P. A hazard of naso-tracheal intubation. *Anaesthesia*. 1978;33:78.
4. Rosen C. Blind nasotracheal intubation in the presence of facial trauma. *J of Emerg Med*. 1997;15:141–145.
5. Goodisson DW, Shaw GM, Snap L. Intracranial intubation in patients with maxillofacial injuries associated with base of skull fractures? *J Trauma*. 2001;50:363–366.
6. Sweeney JM, Lebovitz JJ, Eller JL, Coppens JR, Bucholz RD, Abdulrauf SI. Management of nonmissile penetrating brain injuries: a description of three cases and review of the literature. *Skull Base Rep*. 2011 May;1(1):39–46
7. Kazim SF, Shamim MS, Tahir MZ, Enam SA, Waheed S. Management of penetrating brain injury. *J Emerg Trauma Shock*. 2011; 4(3):395–402.
8. Aarabi B. Traumatic aneurysms of brain due to high velocity missile head wounds. *Neurosurgery*. 1988;22:1056–1063.
9. Haddad FS, Haddad GF, Taha J. Traumatic intracranial aneurysms caused by missiles: their presentation and management. *Neurosurgery*. 1997;28:1–7.

CHAPTER 20

Brain Herniation

A Delayed Complication

Scharukh Jalisi
Samuel J. Rubin
Kevin Wu

THE CASE

A 45-year-old automobile mechanic presented to Otolaryngology clinic with a history of recurrent inverted papilloma (IP). He was originally diagnosed six years prior when he developed a swollen right eye that was thought to be due to a right frontal mucocele. He was treated with intravenous antibiotics and subsequent surgery through a lateral rhinotomy approach/lynch incision where pathology diagnosed IP. In the six years before we met him, he underwent nine procedures for recurrent IP including endoscopic approaches and finally an osteoplastic approach to the frontal sinus. Of note, he had a long history of recurrent sinusitis dating back to childhood and mild diabetes mellitus, type 2. He denied alcohol use, illicit drug use, or cigarette smoking.

He was referred to our tertiary care center for worsening right eye proptosis and abnormal imaging. A recent MRI scan showed a mass extending from the intracranial cavity into the right nasal cavity and ethmoid sinuses with dural enhancement. The lesion was suggestive for an encephalocele. Additionally, another lesion was found in the right frontal sinus extending into the posterior apex of the right orbit (Figure 20–1). A CT scan demonstrated a soft tissue mass within

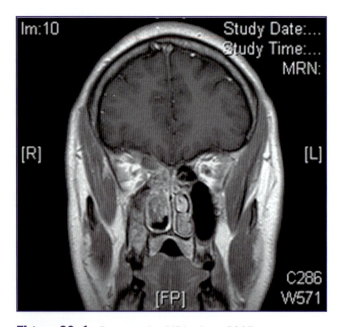

Figure 20–1. Preoperative MRI—June 2007.

the posterior right nasal cavity measuring 2.5 cm × 1.7 cm. A lesion within the right anterior nasal cavity extended into the ethmoid sinus, frontal sinus, and medial right orbit was also identified. Within the orbit, the globe was displaced inferolaterally resulting in proptosis. Additionally, there were focal areas of bony thinning and dehiscence on the right skull base and orbit (Figure 20–2).

In order to eradicate the disease, prevent orbital and intracranial complications from local compression, and reconstruct the defects, a craniofacial resection approach of the mass-occupying lesion was recommended. A multidisciplinary team included a head and neck surgeon, neurosurgeon, and oculoplastic surgeon. The patient was advised of the usual risks of craniofacial resection including infection, bleeding, inadequate healing, persistence or recurrence of tumor, numbness, scarring, visual changes, injury to eye, injury to the facial nerve, cerebrospinal fluid leak, stroke, and death.

A lumbar drain was placed before beginning the resection in anticipation of a high-flow CSF leak. Subsequently, the craniofacial resection was performed without difficulty. Once the bifrontal craniotomy was performed to facilitate access to the anterior skull base, 40 mL of CSF was released from the lumbar drain. The posterior wall of the frontal sinus was taken down and a large mucocele was encountered in the frontal sinus extending into the right orbit and medial wall of the sinus. The tumor was identified and resected followed by

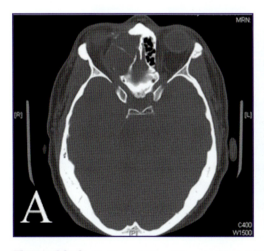
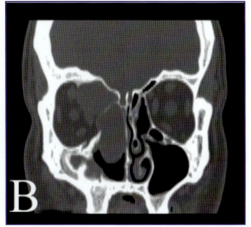

Figure 20–2. **A.** Preoperative CT scan, August 2007—axial image. **B.** Preoperative CT scan, August 2007—coronal image.

reconstruction with a titanium mesh to cover the cribriform defect, AlloDerm to protect the brain from the mesh (Figure 20–3), and a pericranial flap from the left supratrochlear vessels (Figure 20–4). 4-0 nylon sutures were used to close any dural defects. The frontal bone was used for a cranioplasty to cover the skull defect. The patient did not experience any problem throughout the procedure and was extubated at the conclusion of the case. He was admitted to the surgical intensive care unit for monitoring and lumbar drain management.

The patient was initially doing well with intact ocular and neurological function. The lumbar drain was working properly and draining at 10 cc/hour with no evidence of a cerebrospinal fluid leak. However, on the second postoperative day, the patient became difficult to arouse. The lumbar drain was then immediately clamped and a stat CT scan of the brain indicated herniation of the brain at the foramen magnum (!), but no bleeding was evident (Figure 20–5). Upon chart review, it was found that the patient drained off 80 cc of CSF in the hour prior to the stat page.

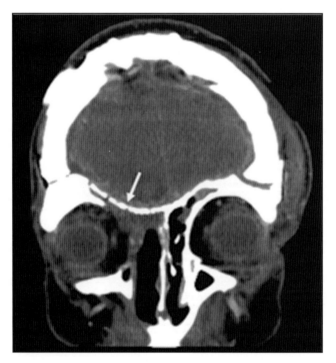

Figure 20–3. Reconstruction of skull base using mesh, pericranial flap, and AlloDerm.

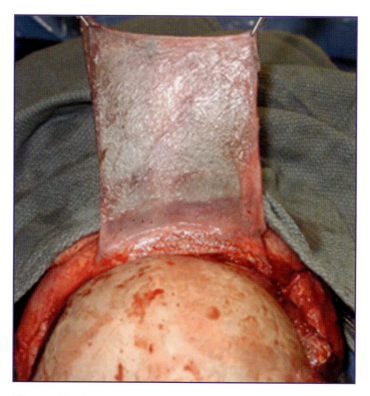

Figure 20–4. Dissected pericranial flap.

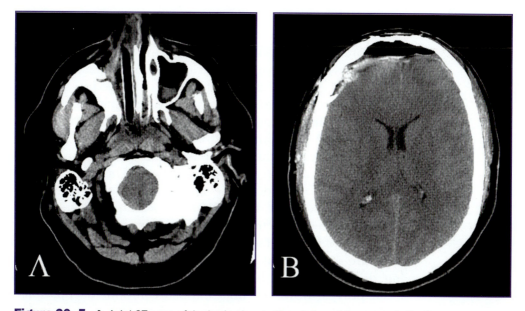

Figure 20–5. A. Axial CT scan of the brain showing herniation of the uncus in the foramen magnum due to rapid loss of cerebrospinal fluid. **B.** The lateral ventricles are effaced.

THIS CASE WAS SCARY BECAUSE

This case was scary because we faced a new, potentially devastating complication that can lead to severe morbidity or even death. There was also concern that the complication may have resulted from an error in patient care that could have been preventable.

THE PATHOLOGY

The tumor was found to be IP of the sinonasal tract with intracranial extension. There were no malignant or invasive features on final pathology. IP is rare with an incidence of 0.2 to 0.6 per 100,000 people and they represent 0.5% to 4% of sinonasal tumors.[1] Furthermore, most patients with IP present in the fifth and sixth decade of life.[1] Intracranial extension of inverted papilloma has been seen in 1.8 to 3% of cases.[2,3] The most common sites of origin for IP include the ethmoid sinus (38%), followed by the maxillary sinus (28%), the sphenoid sinus (14%), the superior turbinate (10%), and the frontal recess (7%).[4] Management of IP includes complete resection to avoid local spread to the intracranial and orbital cavities or, rarely, malignant transformation occurs.[4]

There is variability in the IP recurrence rate in the literature with studies reporting a recurrence rate of 5% to 32%.[5,6] Therefore, it is often necessary to perform multiple surgical procedures over an extended period of time to manage extensive lesions. Some of the key features described in management of IP to minimize recurrence is careful management of the site of tumor attachment, irrespective of tumor size or formal stage.[4] Furthermore, drilling, or completely excising the bone underlying the tumor base rather than mucosal stripping results in a lower rate of recurrence.[7] There is currently a debate whether endoscopic surgical techniques result in a lower recurrence rate than other surgical approaches; however, there are conflicting results in the literature.[4,8]

Some of the risk factors associated with an increased rate of IP are outdoor and industrial occupations, tobacco smoking, drinking alcohol, history of allergic rhinitis, sinusitis, and nasal polyps; however, high exposure indoor occupations, such as a car mechanic, are not associate with increased risk of IP.[9] Additionally, the most common presenting symptoms for inverted papilloma include nasal obstruction, epistaxis, facial pain, and postnasal drip.[1] Although most IP today can be treated with an endoscopic approach, tumor extension into the frontal sinus and orbit are often managed with an external approach because these areas are frequent sites of recurrent disease.[10]

A review of patients with intracranial extension of IP indicated that extradural disease had a survival rate of 86% with an average follow-up of 4.4 years (86% of patients treated with craniofacial resection), while 75% of patients with intradural IP did not survive with an average follow-up of 9.3 months regardless of treatment modality.[11] However, there were no reported recurrences after craniofacial resection with a mean follow-up of 7.9 years.[12]

There are no reported cases of uncal herniation through the foramen magnum resulting from craniofacial resection of the anterior fossa, although a rapid loss of CSF is a known cause of uncal herniation. Some of the complications associated with anterior craniofacial resection include meningitis, cerebrospinal leak, cerebral abscess, and subdural hemorrhage.[13] Whereas the complication associated with resection of IP resection in general include: facial numbness, cerebrospinal fluid leaks, epistaxis, epiphora, and diplopia.[7,14–16]

CASE OUTCOME

The stat head CT scan revealed uncal herniation due to a rapid loss of CSF from the lumbar drain. As soon as the problem was identified, fifty ml of normal saline was infused into the lumbar drain to replace the lost CSF. On postoperative day #3, the patient became arousable with an improved Glasgow Coma Scale of 7 from 3. On postoperative day #5, further improvement was evident with the patient being awake and extubated. The patient was able to ambulate there days later and was discharged to the rehabilitation floor on postoperative day #10. The only persistent defect was a divergent ocular gaze. He was deemed disabled due to diplopia and a right homonymous hemianopia. Fortunately, the patient regained normal vision and intact gaze at 4 months following surgery. The patient subsequently received 5940 cGy of radiation therapy over a 6-week period. He has not required any additional surgical procedures for recurrence of inverted papilloma and the patient is disease free after 8 years of follow-up.

WHAT I LEARNED FROM THIS CASE

What I learned from this case is that the brain herniation was likely a result of a communication lapse between the nursing staff and the multiple services giving orders for management of the lumbar drain. There were slight variations in the orders provided by the two services resulting in confusion. It is necessary to optimize communication between the nursing staff and managing services, and one service alone (either Otolaryngology or Neurosurgery) should manage the lumbar drain. Furthermore, it is crucial to have a well-trained team to diagnose and manage threatening complications such as the one described, including intensivists, nursing, otolaryngologists, neurosurgeons, and neuroradiologists. As a result of this case, our institution instituted a new policy of a single team managing a patient's lumbar drain. I also learned that the brain could recover if problems are diagnosed early, and that compassion and truthful disclosure are essential to patient care.

REFERENCES

1. Harvey RJ, Sheahan PO, Schlosser RJ. Surgical management of benign sinonasal masses. *Otolaryngol Clin North Am.* 2009;42(2): 353–375.
2. Lawson W, Patel ZM. The evolution of management for inverted papilloma: an analysis of 200 cases. *Otolaryngol Head Neck Surg.* 2009;140(3):330–335.
3. Vrabec DP. The inverted Schneiderian papilloma: a 25-year study. *Laryngoscope.* 1994;104(5 Pt 1):582–605.
4. Busquets JM, Hwang PH. Endoscopic resection of sinonasal inverted papilloma: a meta-analysis. *Otolaryngol Head Neck Surg.* 2006;134(3):476–482.
5. Sham CL, Woo JK, Van hasselt CA, Tong MC. Treatment results of sinonasal inverted papilloma: an 18-year study. *Am J Rhinol Allergy.* 2009;23(2):203–211.
6. Suh JD, Chiu AG. What are the surveillance recommendations following resection of sinonasal inverted papilloma? *Laryngoscope.* 2014;124(9):1981–1982.
7. Healy DY, Chhabra N, Metson R, Holbrook EH, Gray ST. Surgical risk factors for recurrence of inverted papilloma. *Laryngoscope.* 2016;126(4): 796–801.
8. Xiao-ting W, Peng L, Xiu-qing W, et al. Factors affecting recurrence of sinonasal inverted papilloma. *Eur Arch Otorhinolaryngol.* 2013;270(4):1349–1353.

9. Sham CL, Lee DL, Van hasselt CA, Tong MC. A case-control study of the risk factors associated with sinonasal inverted papilloma. *Am J Rhinol Allergy*. 2010;24(1):e37–e40.
10. Lawson W, Kaufman MR, Biller HF. Treatment outcomes in the management of inverted papilloma: an analysis of 160 cases. *Laryngoscope*. 2003;113(9):1548–1556.
11. Vural E, Suen JY, Hanna E. Intracranial extension of inverted papilloma: an unusual and potentially fatal complication. *Head Neck*. 1999;21(8):703–706.
12. Wright EJ, Chernichenko N, Ocal E, Moliterno J, Bulsara KR, Judson BL. Benign inverted papilloma with intracranial extension: prognostic factors and outcomes. *Skull Base Rep*. 2011;1(2):145–150.
13. Dias FL, Sá GM, Kligerman J, et al. Complications of anterior craniofacial resection. *Head Neck*. 1999;21(1):12–20.
14. Lombardi D, Tomenzoli D, Buttà L, et al. Limitations and complications of endoscopic surgery for treatment for sinonasal inverted papilloma: a reassessment after 212 cases. *Head Neck*. 2011;33(8):1154–1161.
15. Kaza S., Capasso R., Casiano R.R. Endoscopic resection of inverted papilloma: University of Miami Experience. *Am. J. Rhinol*. 2003;17(4):185–190.
16. Castelnuovo P, Pagella F, Semino L, De bernardi F, Delù G. Endoscopic treatment of the isolated sphenoid sinus lesions. *Eur Arch Otorhinolaryngol*. 2005;262(2):142–147.

SECTION 5

Vascular Injuries

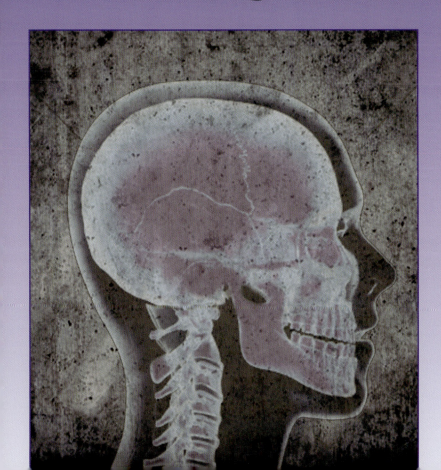

CHAPTER 21

Aberrant Carotid

A Bloody Myringotomy

Yehia Mohammed Ashry
Dennis S. Poe

Myringotomy and tympanostomy tube insertion is one of the most commonly performed operations among all surgical procedures, and significant complications are rare. Vascular complications are exceedingly rare and, understandably, occur completely unexpectedly. It is hard to imagine a worse nightmare than to have a routine and straightforward procedure, in an otherwise healthy patient, suddenly deteriorate into a life-threatening and potentially catastrophic crisis.

THE CASE

A 7-year-old female presented with a recurrence of bilateral otitis media with effusion after having undergone uneventful bilateral myringotomy and tympanostomy tube insertions on a previous occasion. On the present day, she was happy, cooperative, and planning to have the tubes placed while she was awake and accompanied by her father in the operating room. The left myringotomy and tube insertion proceeded uneventfully. On the right side, upon making the myringotomy in the anterior-inferior quadrant, there was "extreme bleeding" that her father later reported had hit the ceiling. The surgeon responded quickly to control the massive bleeding, packing the external auditory canal with Gelfoam and Sepragel (hyaluronic nasal packing), rapidly, but carefully, followed by placement of an external mastoid dressing.

A second attack of bleeding occurred a short time afterward, despite the packing in place, and she was transported to our tertiary referral center. En route, she had a moderate amount of bleeding (≈ 30 mL). On arrival, she was awake, alert, oriented, comfortable, and without any active bleeding. Her vital signs were stable. There was a blood-soaked mastoid dressing over her ear, and she had no neurological deficits. Computed tomography angiography with IV contrast was obtained and showed bilaterally aberrant internal carotid arteries (Figure 21–1). They were of normal caliber but displaced posteriorly and laterally into the middle ear with dehiscence of the bony covering. In the absence of any further bleeding, she was admitted for close observation, and blood type and cross-match were ordered.

At 01:00 that night she developed sudden significant bleeding (≈ 100 mL) for which she was transferred immediately to the operating room (OR) for possible emergency exploration and packing. While waiting in the OR, the interventional

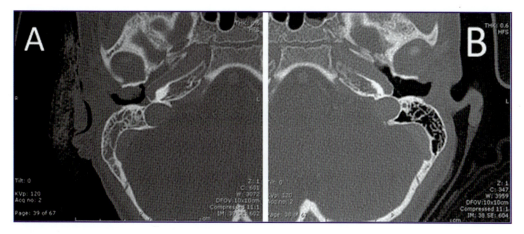

Figure 21–1. Computed tomography angiography with IV contrast showed bilaterally aberrant internal carotid arteries.

radiology team was called in and she was transferred to the interventional radiology suite as soon as the team arrived.

During transportation, there was another episode of brisk bleeding (≈100 mL) which was controlled with external pressure over the external auditory meatus. Angiography showed a 3-mm pseudoaneurysm of the petrous segment of the aberrant right internal carotid artery (ICA). There was excellent collateral circulation through the anterior communicating artery from the left ICA and from the right posterior communicating artery from the vertebra-basilar circulation. The blood loss from the ear continued sporadically throughout the angiography to total about 300 mL. The senior author remained with the patient throughout the diagnostic procedure.

A difficult decision process then ensued as how to best manage her life-threatening situation. Continued observation was no longer an option given the repeated and increasingly severe bleeds. The injury was located between curves in the ICA that would not permit placement of endovascular stents. Occlusion of the right ICA seemed to be the only option, but it presented an extremely disquieting situation for the interventional radiologist, who had not been previously prepared to consider the risks of complete occlusion in an otherwise healthy child. Occlusion could be performed surgically, but would require hours of additional time before achieving adequate surgical exposure to safely ligate or occlude the vessel. Open suture repair of the vessel could be technically feasible, but would require a large skull base approach that would leave her with an overclosed ear canal and conductive hearing loss. After calling and waking up some neurovascular surgeons for additional opinions, a consensus was achieved to proceed with endovascular occlusion of the vessel.

Occlusion of her right ICA was accomplished proximal and distal to the affected segment by angiographic coiling with a wire embolization coil. She was admitted to the pediatric intensive care unit, anticoagulated on heparin, and her follow-up was unremarkable without any further bleeding or neurological sequelae. She stayed for 3 days in the hospital with uneventful observation and was discharged home.

THE SCARY CASE CONTINUES

At her postoperative follow-up 1 month later, otoscopy revealed that her embolization coil was extruding out from the ICA and slightly tenting the tympanic membrane. At 3 months follow-up there was further extrusion of the coil and further tenting of the tympanic membrane (TM) to the point of risking extrusion through the TM (Figures 21–2A and B). This presented a new and difficult challenge. A search of the literature failed to find any previously reported such cases. In phone consultations with neurotology colleagues, no one had ever encountered this situation. The interventional radiologist cautioned against any manipulation of the embolization coil out of concern that the occlusion could be disrupted. Trimming the coil was not an option as it would risk displacing the coil. We finally decided to reinforce the TM with a cartilage graft to prevent penetration through the TM and hope that the rigidity of the graft would prevent further extrusion of the coil.

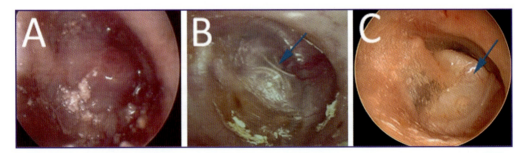

Figure 21–2. A–B. At 3 months follow-up there was further extrusion of the coil and further tenting of the tympanic membrane to the point of risking extrusion (*blue arrow is the coil*). **C.** Eight years later, oto-microscopic examination shows a well-healed graft and the embolization coil is not visible (*blue arrow*).

A transcanal tympanoplasty was performed, placing a tragal cartilage graft medial to the tympanic membrane. Eight years later, she continues to do well. Oto-microscopic examination shows a well-healed graft (Figure 21–2C), and the embolization coil is not visible. She has a stable mild conductive hearing loss (Figure 21–3). The aberrant ICA on the opposite left ear remains visible and unchanged.

DISCUSSION

An aberrant carotid artery is thought to be an exceptionally rare developmental anomaly of the stapedial artery, or its branch, that persist to give rise to an ICA that takes an unusually lateral course and brings it into a vulnerable position within the middle ear.[1] If the bony covering over the vessel is dehiscent, the vessel is exposed to injury during middle ear surgery and misguided attempts to biopsy a vascular lesion of uncertain etiology.[1-3]

There are only a few reports of aberrant ICAs into the middle ear. Windfuhr[4] reviewed the existing case series to summarize the findings in a total of 86 cases: 26 (30%) patients were men, 59 (69%) were women, and it occurred bilaterally in 13 (15%) individuals. The mean age was 22.6 years old (range 9 months to 72 years, SD 17.8 years). The diagnosis was made with bleeding from accidental injury of the ICA in 36 cases

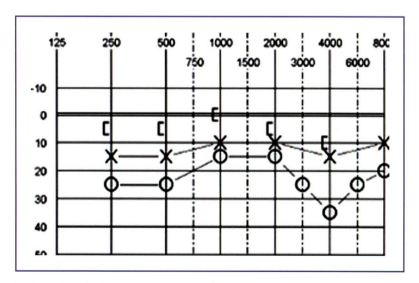

Figure 21–3. Postoperative audiogram shows a stable mild conductive hearing loss.

(42%) during tympanotomy, myringotomy, or biopsy,[4] suggesting that the aberrancy is frequently unsuspected.

Clinical diagnosis of the aberrant ICA is challenging as it may be asymptomatic or presenting with nonspecific symptoms such as pulsatile tinnitus, aural fullness, or conductive hearing loss. Otoscopic examination of the ear may find a reddish-blue mass in the anterior-inferior quadrant of the middle ear, and it may slightly tent up the tympanic membrane laterally. The vessel may sometimes impinge on the umbo of the malleus. The examination may be normal if the artery is obscured by effusion or scarring in the tympanic membrane.[1]

The differential diagnosis of a vascular mass within the middle ear may include ICA aneurysm, high jugular bulb, otosclerosis, paraganglioma (glomus tumor) or other neoplasm, arteriovenous malformation, and other vascular malformations.[5] Evaluation of a vascular mass within the middle ear should always be done by imaging studies and biopsy can be considered if the diagnosis remains uncertain after ruling out aberrancy of the ICA or jugular bulb. Imaging studies may include high-resolution computerized tomography (HRCT) or magnetic resonance imaging (MRI) to look for vascular lesions. Injection of IV contrast enhances the clarity of vascular anatomy in both studies. CT angiography or magnetic resonance angiography is important in assessing vascular supply, injury, and collateral circulation,[6] and angiography remains the "gold standard" for delineating the most details of vascular anatomy and collateral circulation.

When a vascular lesion is discovered during middle ear examination and it does not appear to be a thin-walled aneurysm, a 27-gauge needle can be introduced into the mass to see if blood can be easily aspirated. If so, it is likely a major vessel. If it remains uncertain if it is venous or arterial, aspiration and blood gas analysis can be performed.[7]

After establishing the diagnosis, a patient should be informed about this condition and the risk of catastrophic bleeding with any middle ear procedure such as myringotomy, tympanotomy, or biopsy. An aberrant ICA can simply be followed conservatively, but for patients with persistent, disturbing pulsatile tinnitus or pulsatile pressure symptoms, surgical management can be offered by covering the displaced artery by a piece of cartilage or bone.[8]

When accidental injury of an aberrant vessel occurs intraoperatively, the surgeon should place a finger over the external auditory meatus tightly and take a moment to collect their astonished wits. This is a frightening and surprising event that requires a rapid, but rational response. The surgeon should call for the necessary large 7 or 9 French suction and packing materials. If the head is elevated at all, it should be placed flat or slightly into Trendelenburg position to avoid aspiration of an air embolus if a venous bleed is suspected. A jugular bulb will bleed impressively but not under significant pressure, and it is readily controlled with moderate packing using absorbable materials such as Gelfoam or Surgicel against the injured vessel so that it will not have to be removed at a later time. These materials get caught in a suction, so a portion of cotton between the suction catheter and the packing material allows the suction to clear blood while advancing the packing in place. A venous bleed will stop promptly, and the cotton can be removed within 5 minutes. If the bleed is arterial, it will be under significant pressure and may be difficult to control. Stopping the bleed is a lifesaving maneuver and the external auditory canal should be packed in a similar fashion with Gelfoam, Surgicel, or whatever is necessary to stop the bleed. Gauze strip packing can be effective. The packing must be done as firmly as necessary to control the bleeding, knowing that excessive pressure may damage the structures of the ear. External compression by a mastoid dressing may be helpful to stabilize the packing within the external auditory canal. Once control of bleeding has been achieved, immediate interventional angiography is indicated to establish a diagnosis, existence of collateral circulation, and definitive treatment options.

For a small injury that was readily controlled, observation may be considered if hemostasis continues, leaving the packing within the external auditory canal for 7 to 10 days[3] in order to allow healing of the lacerated artery. It should be kept in mind that delayed onset of bleeding has been reported as long as 39 days after carotid injury.[2] Consideration should be made about removal of the packing in the operating room. Further follow-up is necessary for observation of recurrent bleeding or development of pseudo-aneurysm.

If bleeding fails to stop after packing or recurs after removal of the packs, occlusion[2] or ligation of the ICA should be urgently arranged after angiography to confirm sufficient collateral circulation. Occlusion of the ICA can be done using balloon or coiling embolization by an interventional radiologist or a neurosurgeon. Sacrifice of the ICA is a procedure of last resort to avoid the possible neurological sequelae. After ICA occlusion or ligation, patients should be followed up closely in the hospital and after their discharge for recurrent bleeding or neurological complications.

The rate of complications from injury of the aberrant ICA or its management by packing, occlusion, or ligation is significantly high at 9/36 (25%) of the cases that presented with intraoperative bleeding in the review by Windfuhr. The complications included pseudoaneurysm, Horner syndrome, facial weakness, conductive hearing loss, deafness, vertigo, hemiparesis (4/9 cases), aphasia (3/9 cases), or even death.[1,2] It is noteworthy that 11% of the 36 cases that presented with intraoperative bleeding suffered major cerebrovascular injuries.

Extrusion of the embolization coil into the middle ear was a minor complication that occured in our case and also in another report by Chow et al.[9] Options for management of coil extrusion are observation if it is stable or placing a piece of cartilage between the occluded ICA with its extruded coil and the tympanic membrane in case of progressive extrusion.[10]

Clearly, maintaining awareness of the possibility for vascular lesions in any ear and early recognition of such lesions to prevent injury is recommended. When an injury occurs, it becomes a complex problem that requires a team effort, but the surgeon must remain as the captain of the team to lead in helping everyone, including the patient and family, through the difficult decisions and challenging procedures.

ASK THE EXPERT: Anthony Abeln, JD

What are the legal risks of allowing family members in the OR for induction of anesthesia (pediatrics) or to watch the surgery (colleagues)?

Generally, for a host of reasons, only the parent or guardian of a pediatric patient is allowed in for a surgery, and usually then only until anesthetic induction. One critical issue is to follow your institutional policy regarding informing a patient (or their guardians/parents) well in advance about who is allowed in during a procedure and when. Early communication can protect against an uncomfortable and even hostile surgical day. Generally, family members and friends who are colleagues should not be present during the surgery as they place increased pressure on the surgeon and provide an unhelpful presence should there be a complication.

The classic cases of medical malpractice emerge when what a family member believed was a relatively benign operation faces a severe complication ("This was only a knee surgery," or "she was supposed be out after a few hours!"). Our doctor above focuses on one of the key issues in medicine—communication! Communicating with patients and their families is a critical part of not only best practices, but is also a way to inoculate yourself from a potential lawsuit when a complication does occur.

> It does help family members, as well, to know that there is a point person whom they can reach out to with questions or concerns; there are times when they approach a fellow or a resident for information, don't receive the full picture they feel that they need, and then doubt that anyone has a full view of their family member's picture. Communication is key!

REFERENCES

1. Hunt JT, Andrews TM. Management of aberrant internal carotid artery injuries in children. *Am J Otolaryngol.* 2000;21:50–54.
2. Brodish BN, Woolley AL. Major vascular injuries in children undergoing myringotomy for tube placement. *Am J Otolaryngol.* 1999;20:46–50.
3. Oates JW, McAuliffe W, Coates HLC. Management of pseudo-aneurysm of a lateral aberrant internal carotid artery. *Int J Pediatr Otorhinolaryngol.* 1997;42:73–79.
4. Windfuhr JP. Aberrant internal carotid artery in the middle ear. *Ann Otol Rhinol Laryngol.* 2004;113:1–16.
5. Steffen TN. Vascular anomalites of the middle ear. *Laryngoscope* 1968;78:171.
6. Lo WW, Solti-Bohman LG, McElveen JT. Aberrant carotid artery: radiologic diagnosis with emphasis on high-resolution computed tomography. *Radiographics.* 1985;5:985.
7. Anand VK, Casano PJ, Flaiz RA. Diagnosis and treatment of the carotid artery in the middle ear. *Otolaryngol Head Neck Surg.* 1991;105:743.
8. Glasscock ME, Dickins JRE, Jackson CG, Wiet RJ. Vascular anomalies of the middle ear. *Laryngoscope.* 1980;90:77–88.
9. Chow MW, Chan DTM, Boet R, Poon WS, Sung JKK, Yu SCH. Extrusion of a coil from the internal carotid artery through the middle ear. *Hong Kong Medical Journal = Xianggang yi xue za zhi.* 2004;10:215.
10. Leuin SC, Handwerker J, Rabinov JD, Poe DS. Carotid laceration during myringotomy. *Otolaryngol Head Neck Surg.* 2009;140: 946–947.

CHAPTER 22

Radiation Therapy for Laryngeal Cancer

"Organ Preservation"

Jonathan C. Simmonds
Elie Rebeiz

THE CASE

A 49-year-old patient underwent radiation therapy for a T2 N0 M0 squamous cell carcinoma of the larynx. The decision for primary radiation therapy rather than surgical resection was made by the patient after appropriate tumor board discussion and meetings with both medical and surgical specialties. Six year later, he presented to our medical center for hemoptysis. At that time he was deemed free of disease. While in the emergency department, he had a severe episode of hemoptysis that required transfusion of 4 units of packed red blood cells, and he was admitted to the intensive care unit.

Shortly after admission, he sustained an acute stroke that resulted in unilateral upper and lower extremity weakness. Workup revealed an embolus from a carotid pseudoaneurysm. The sentinel bleed from the carotid artery resulted in a rare complication of embolic stroke. He underwent a successful embolization of the pseudoaneurysm with a coil placement and a stent from the common carotid to the proximal end of the internal carotid bypassing the pseudoaneurysm (Figure 22–1). Radiation therapy is a known risk factor for developing a carotid blowout with hemoptysis as a potential presenting symptom of a sentinel bleed. All sentinel bleeds are scary, but . . .

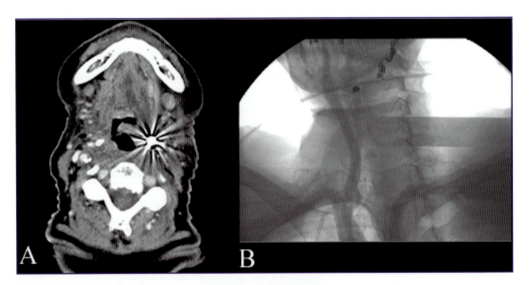

Figure 22–1. A. Neck CT scan prior to the surgery revealed an occluded left CCA with a coil in place and causing artifact that limits detail of the area surrounding the carotid. **B.** Plain x-ray reveals a stent in the common carotid and internal carotid arteries.

THE SCARY CASE CONTINUES

Eighteen months later, the patient presented to the Otolaryngology clinic with recurrent intractable aspiration pneumonias despite being J-tube and tracheotomy dependent. The hopes of "organ preservation" with radiation therapy were not realized as his airway patency, swallowing mechanism, and voice had minimal function. Possible options were discussed including laryngotracheal separation and total laryngectomy. A decision was made to proceed with a narrow-field laryngectomy in order to prevent further aspiration pneumonias.

This case presented numerous challenges because of the many risks in performing a narrow field laryngectomy in a cachectic patient with multiple aspiration pneumonias, a prior stroke, in the setting of radiated neck and larynx, history of an impending carotid blowout syndrome previously managed with embolization and stenting. However, the alternative of not intervening would certainly result in a poor outcome with continued aspiration and malnutrition.

GETTING SCARIER IN THE OPERATING ROOM

The narrow-field laryngectomy proceeded with induction of anesthesia and exposure of the larynx. Besides the usual fibrosis seen in the irradiated neck, the intraoperative findings were surprising and concerning: upon opening the pharynx, there was an unusual foreign body. The embolization coil had migrated through the medial wall of the left common carotid into the hypopharynx (Figure 22–2). The severity of the situation

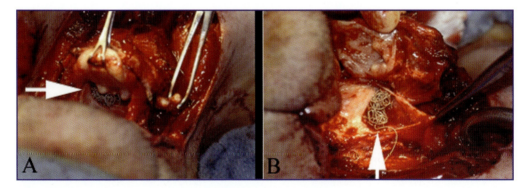

Figure 22–2. A–B. Intraoperative findings during narrow-field laryngectomy. There is an exposed right carotid artery stent, a disintegrated common carotid artery, and a coil (*white arrows*) eroding into the hypopharynx.

dawned on us. At this stage, many intraoperative decisions had to be made:

1. How to manage the coil: Should we remove it? If we do, will the carotid artery bleed, or would emboli be transmitted to the cerebral vasculature and worsen his neurologic deficit?
2. How to manage the carotid stump: ligate the carotid or perform a bypass with vascular surgery?
3. How to close the hypopharynx in an irradiated field: radial forearm free flap, pectoralis major flap, or perform primary closure?

In order to manage the extruding coil and the carotid artery, we obtained an intraoperative vascular surgery consult. The decision was made to cross-clamp and suture ligate the common carotid. The extruding coil was carefully removed without any bleeding.

The second challenge was how to close the hypopharynx of this poorly nourished man, in a radiated field. Knowing that the risk of fistula formation is high, the question was should the pharynx be closed primarily, with a forearm free flap or with a pectoralis major flap? In order to minimize operative time, we decided against using a pedicled or free flap because we felt there was enough hypopharyngeal mucosa to close the neo-pharynx primarily.

WHAT WE LEARNED FROM THIS CASE

Managing complications associated with radiation therapy to the head and neck is complex: one should expect the unexpected especially when complications involve the carotid artery. Radiation damage can weaken the walls of the artery which caused a pseudoaneurysm in our patient. A coil used for embolization of the pseudoaneurysm can eventually migrate and extrude.

There have been many reports of endovascular stents migrating and extruding, thus leaving the common carotid artery exposed to air in a nonsterile field.[1] Chang et al[2] reported a case of carotid blowout syndrome with large area of soft tissue necrosis and ulceration surrounding the stent grafts caused "floating" of left carotid artery. Chang et al[3] also reported a stroke, re-bleeding, delayed thrombosis, and formation of brain abscesses after embolization of the carotid artery. Several reports described migration of the coil through the anterolateral cervical skin[4] into the pharynx[5] and hypopharynx.[6] Perhaps the most important lesson of this case was that dealing with serious and unexpected complications in the operating room requires a thorough understanding of your patient's history to fully understand the pathophysiological changes that lead to an emergency situation.

One of the most important lessons learned in this case was that dealing with serious and unexpected complications in the operating room requires a thorough understanding of your patient's history and of the pathophysiological changes that lead to the emergent situation. In addition, care providers should always follow the golden rule of *asking the expert*. In some cases, the expert is a senior, more experienced surgeon in the same specialty, or a consultant such as a vascular surgeon in this case.

CASE OUTCOME

Fortunately, the postoperative course was uneventful. There was no bleeding and there were no further neurologic deficits; the neo-pharynx healed well. The patient was discharged 6 days later and was able to resume oral intake 2 weeks later. He no longer suffered from aspiration, but voice rehabilitation was required.

CONCLUSION

Carotid blowout syndrome is one of the most dreaded complications of radiation therapy with high mortality and morbidity rates. There are a variety of clinical presentations, including hemoptysis and stroke. Emergency surgical ligation is sometimes required as a lifesaving procedure, and in recent years, endovascular therapeutic techniques have been developed to avoid surgery but are subject to complications. Endovascular imaging helps primarily in obtaining angiographic findings such as the patency of the vessel and presence of emboli and in determining the best course of action.

Successful outcomes are possible if the clinicians maintain a *high index of suspicion and take immediate action*.

REFERENCES

1. Simental A, Johnson J, Horowitz M. Delayed complications of endovascular stenting for carotid blowout. *Am J Otolaryngol.* 2003;24:417–419.
2. Chang FC, Luo CB, Lirng JF, Guo WY, Wu HM, Teng MM, Chang CY. Complications of carotid blowout syndrome in patients with head and neck cancers treated by covered stents. *Interv Neuroradiol.* 2008 Nov;14(suppl 2):29–33.
3. Chang FC, Lirng JF, Luo CB, Guo WY, Teng MM, Tai SK, Chang CY. Carotid blowout syndrome in patients with head-and-neck cancers: reconstructive management by self-expandable stent-grafts. *AJNR Am J Neuroradiol.* 2007 Jan;28(1):181–188.
4. Collignon FP, Friedman JA, Piepgras DG, et al. Transcutaneous coil, stent, and balloon migration following endovascular treatment of a cervical carotid artery aneurysm. Case illustration. *J Neurosurg.* 2003;98:1135.
5. Lin HW, Tierney HT, Richmon JD, et al. Extrusion of embolization coils through the carotid artery in a radiated neck. *Auris Nasus Larynx.* 2010;37:390–393.
6. Iguchi H, Takayama M, Kusuki M, et al. Transmucosal coil migration after endovascular management for carotid artery pseudoaneurysm: a late complication. *Acta Otolaryngol.* 2007;127:447–448.

CHAPTER 23

Helicopter Flight

A Scary Post-Tonsillectomy Bleed

Edward F. Caldwell
Hani Ibrahim

THE CASE

Jane is a 17-year-old red-haired, moderately overweight high school senior who presented to our local emergency room with bright red hemoptysis 7 days after tonsillectomy at a different facility. Her tonsils were removed for recurrent production of tonsilliths and snoring, with no history of recurrent tonsillitis or peritonsillar abscess. There was no personal or family history of bleeding abnormalities. Her postoperative course had been uneventful, with the expected moderate odynophagia. Her food and fluid intake had been adequate. On initial evaluation, while actively suctioning bright red blood from her oropharynx, she reported that bleeding started when she felt "something" in her throat which she cleared vigorously. She generally appeared healthy, well hydrated, and her vital signs were normal. Her exam revealed a large clot filling her right tonsillar fossa, with active bright red oozing blood coming around the clot.

Her mother was a pediatric intensive care unit (ICU) nurse, and she elected to have the tonsillectomy performed at a tertiary care center that was 2 hours away. Her mother had seen post-tonsil bleeding and was familiar with the usual treatment needed. While she had elected for care elsewhere for the tonsillectomy, she recognized the urgency of bleeding and agreed to proceed with exam under anesthesia with control of bleeding at our local hospital where tonsillectomy is routinely performed.

The patient was taken to the operating room, where appropriate monitoring was established, IV access secured, and supplemental oxygen provided. She continued to self-suction blood. There was an experienced anesthesiologist, an experienced otolaryngologist, a circulating nurse, and a scrub technologist present for the start of the case at 11:30 PM.

Because of the ongoing active bleeding, a rapid sequence induction was planned with cricoid pressure to decrease the risk of aspiration. As deep sedation was established with Propofol, without paralysis, the patient developed more active and brisk bleeding. Blood was pooling in the oropharynx preventing visualization of the larynx. There were multiple attempts by the anesthesiologist at intubation that failed because of the inability to visualize the vocal cords around a large tongue and clots. Two suctions were used with repeated intubation using a glide-scope video intubation system. The larynx could not be visualized!

The patient's oxygen saturations progressively fell into the lower 70s, when a third hand with suction appeared . . .

the patient's, and she began to self-suction and speak with immediate resolution of her hypoxia! She was brought to a sitting position while self-suctioning smaller amounts of bright red blood and able to speak. The anesthesiologist and the otolaryngologist appeared pale while the patient had good skin color.

Now what? We went from a very unstable situation to a stable situation, but the problem has not been resolved. She had a clot in the tonsillar fossa that could release anytime and result in airway obstruction. The attending surgeon left the operating room to inform her mother of the events and discuss the next steps and options. Her mother was told about the extreme difficulty in intubation with life-threatening hypoxia, something that she was very familiar with having worked in the pediatric ICU.

There was no doubt that the bleeding required control, and the airway needed to be secured. Given the difficulties encountered, the safest way to establish an airway was through a tracheostomy. Since she had stable vital signs and the ability to protect her airway, local anesthesia was the preferred method. There was no possibility that the anesthesiologist who just encountered a near-death would repeat a rapid-sequence induction.

It was now near 1:00 AM, and another option was proposed. Her exam showed that the clot was essentially unchanged with ongoing mild oozing and her post-"procedure" hematocrit was minimally decreased. Her mother was offered transfer to the tertiary care center where the tonsillectomy was performed. Her mother did not like the idea of awake tracheostomy and elected to return to Boston. Since it was felt this should be done as quickly as possible, the Life Flight helicopter was summoned. The patient was transferred to recovery room with the entire team present.

The Life Flight team arrived 40 minutes later. She was evaluated by a flight nurse and a paramedic who had significant experience with life-threatening transports. After hearing the situation and examining her, they stated that transport could only happen if the patient's airway were secured. However, the attending anesthesiologist pointed out that the patient had a life-threatening bout of hypoxia during the first attempt and refused intubation. The attending otolaryngologist stated that he would recommend tracheotomy be performed, which the mother and patient refused.

Multiple conference calls were held with the flight director for Life Flight, an attending anesthesiologist at the accepting facility, and the attending otolaryngologist. After 1 hour of negotiating, we were deadlocked—the anesthesiologist would not intubate, the flight nurse would not transport, and the patient's family would not agree to a tracheostomy. Yet the patient was still oozing from around a large clot that could release at any time. No one wanted to accept the liability of a possible death from airway obstruction in a young patient.

THE SOLUTION

At 2:30 AM, a sidebar discussion was held with the mother and her patient explaining the issues and the risks. It was proposed that the mother sign a release from liability form for the Life Flight, stating that they could not be held accountable if she were to lose her airway during the flight. Fortunately, the bleeding had subsided with a smaller clot present. The Life Flight accepted the release and agreed to transport across the bay to the tertiary care center. As expected, the transport was uneventful. She was taken to the OR on arrival, successfully intubated without difficulty, and a very small area of oozing controlled with electrocautery. She was discharged home the following day to complete her recovery.

THIS CASE WAS SCARY BECAUSE

A perfect storm of events can result in a routine case becoming extremely stressful and life threatening. A moderately overweight healthy young woman with active bleeding and clots becomes an anesthesiologist's nightmare when alone overnight. Off-hour OR procedures limit the number of experienced minds and hands to help, although it may not have changed the situation. Airway bleeding cases are by their nature never "routine." Multiple anesthesiologists may be necessary and are usually present with difficult airway cases during peak hours. It also can be helpful to have 2 otolaryngologists present, one to assist anesthesia, the other to prepare for a surgical airway. Obviously, in the vast majority of cases there will be no need for the added personnel, but when it goes poorly, it does so quickly.

Glide scopes have become a mainstay of assistance in the intubation of difficult airways, yet they become useless if blood covers their lens. Some institutions have the luxury of multiple prepared glide scopes should there be a need. Alternately, staff should be trained and anticipate the need to rapidly clean the lens of glide scopes in such situations.

The Life Flight transfer was a "Catch 22"—we were at risk with transfer, we were at risk without transfer. All transfers for "airway obstruction" to a center with a higher level of acuity offer this unique problem. The accepting institution always recommends securing the airway prior to transport, yet the difficult airway is the indication for transfer. There is increased risk with either decision, and the clinician who had the advantage of examining the patient is often in a better position to make these difficult decisions.

Life Flight routinely transfers critically ill patients with compromised airways from the field with hesitation, yet with an elective transport, they were unwilling to transfer. An "airway" specialist could ask, "Why don't you secure the airway prior to transfer" for all trauma patients with compromised airways, but the level of risk with an elective case is much greater than that with a trauma situation where there is a greater cushion for adverse outcomes.

WHAT I LEARNED FROM THIS CASE

We are all part of the same team, including the anesthesiologist, the med-flight team, the accepting institution physicians, the patient, and the family. When presented with a dilemma, all parties should be included in the decision with risks shared among those involved. This case could have had a much worse outcome, had the patient had a severe bleed in the OR, the ED, or the helicopter. Having the patient and her mother involved in all decisions was essential to achieving the good outcome.

Second, when dealing with an airway problem, nothing is ever routine. I have learned to be prepared for the worst. There is often more assistance available during the day than at night, but the clinical scenario of an emergency requires that we do our best with the available resources. There is usually someone else you can call for help if time allows, and you should never be afraid to ask for help.

ASK THE EXPERT: Anthony Abeln, JD

Can I refuse a transfer?
The Emergency Medical Treatment and Labor Act (EMTALA) was put in place where there was a concern by Congress that "hospitals were 'dumping' patients who were unable to pay, by either refusing to provide emergency medical treatment or transferring patients before their conditions were stabilized." *Eberhardt v. City of Los Angeles*, 62 F.3d 1253, 1255 (9th Cir.1995). The law also has a "reverse

dumping" provision, to protect against hospitals from refusing to accept transfers where it has specialized capabilities to help a patient. See *St. Anthony Hosp. v. U.S. Dept. of Health and Human Services*, 309 F.3d 680 (10th Cir).

At the center of the transferor's EMTALA responsibility is that the patient needs to be stabilized before transport. But by whom? Should the hospital have sent a physician along with the Life Flight team? Should any airway obstruction transfer be accompanied by a physician? Would securing the airway be riskier for a particular patient? Medical judgment, as noted by the author, is the key—is the patient stable—that is, is it reasonable that the patient's condition won't deteriorate during transfer.

Further, remember all of the other issues that arise out of transfers—have the patient's needs and history been sufficiently communicated? Are all of the proper records (CTs, MRIs, plain films, etc) transferred with the patient? Imagine a scary case where a key study was not included with a transferred patient, and there was an adverse outcome!

Of course, a physician (and likely the hospital, too) can face potential discipline for an inappropriate transfer—whether patient dumping, reverse dumping, or by a problematic transfer process. Enforcement of such inappropriate care is often done through a department safety officer, the department chair, or a complaint to the State Board of Registration in Medicine. In reality, these cases often have 2 sides to the story and are not straightforward in determining whether care was inappropriate.

Finally, while physicians and hospitals are bound to EMTALA, medical negligence in a civil court typically cannot be claimed until there is a treating relationship between the physician and patient. Where a physician refuses transfer, a professional relationship has not yet been established, so the normal medical negligence paradigm might not apply. However, a claimant will certainly try to raise other theories on the periphery of medical malpractice to allege that the refusing doctor failed to act reasonably under the circumstances. The scope of that duty can differ across jurisdictions.

CHAPTER 24

Sentinel Bleed

The Saturday Night Bleeder

Barry J. Benjamin
Namita R. Murthy

THE CASE

A 66-year-old man presented to a colleague for a right neck mass. He underwent workup for malignancy including imaging, endoscopy, and biopsies that did not reveal a malignancy. He had a history of undergoing a Thorotrast carotid angiogram approximately 15 years earlier. He agreed to excisional biopsy.

The surgery was not routine. There was extensive fibrosis that made dissection of the mass very difficult. The mass was encasing the carotid artery and with the extensive fibrosis, the artery was entered during dissection. Carotid ligation was required to control the bleeding. This was the first scary part of the case, but the patient did not develop any neurological deficits postoperatively. Pathology revealed extensive fibrosis with dense aggregates of dark-brown refractile material and chronic inflammatory cells focally present. Brown, refractile granules are characteristic of Thorotrast.

I was on-call for my colleague over the weekend when the floor nurse called for bleeding. The patient was 3-days status postexcision. He was immediately taken to the operating room (OR) for exploration. As I opened the wound, blood began to well-up from under the clavicle. Where was it coming from? I have never treated a bleed from under the clavicle. I was only able to control the bleeding by reaching into the upper mediastinum and applying digital pressure. I could not remove my finger! I could not see where the bleeding was coming from! I was alone in an OR with an emergency on a Saturday night!

There is always someone you can call for help. I called the thoracic surgeon and waited for the chief resident and attending to open the chest and stop the bleeding. The bleeding was coming from the junction of the innominate artery and the aorta. They were able to repair the vessel and close the chest without difficulty. The patient made an uneventful recovery and was discharged after 1 week.

WHY DID THIS HAPPEN?

Thorotrast is a thorium dioxide suspension that was used as a contrast dye until the early 1950s.[1,2] It was radioactive with a half-life of 22 years. It was discontinued because it was carcinogenic and caused extensive fibrosis including nerve weakness and vascular obliteration. Vascular erosion and hemorrhage are secondary to Thorotrast extravasation at the time of injection with long-term exposure to the radiation.

THIS CASE WAS SCARY BECAUSE

I usually do not deal with bleeding from the great vessels. There was a major complication on a patient whom I was covering for on the weekend. I was alone on a Saturday night, and I wasn't sure if I would be able to find help in time.

WHAT I LEARNED FROM THIS CASE

It is never too soon to call for help. Don't be afraid of reaching out to colleagues sooner rather than later as you don't know how long it will take for help to arrive.

Suspect a sentinel bleed from a major vessel. Life-threatening bleeds often start as a small trickle. The clinical scenario of bleeding in the neck or oral cavity in a patient who underwent surgery or has cancer should alert clinicians to the sentinel bleed.

Although it is a rare occurrence, consider Thorotrast toxicity in older patients with unexplained or undefined neck mass with fibrosis.

CAROTID BLOWOUT SYNDROME

Carotid blowout syndrome (CBS) is a dreaded and often fatal complication of head and neck malignancies. The incidence of CBS ranges from 2.6% to 4.3% after radical surgical excision and radiation therapy for head and neck cancer. The reported mortality of CBS is 40% with an associated morbidity up to 60%. Disrupting the vaso vasorum blood supply to the carotid artery by carotid isolation and exposure leads to weakening of the vessel wall with possible rupture.

Risk factors for developing CBS after neck surgery include direct involvement of recurrent tumor, pharyngocutaneous fistula, deep neck abscess, or radiation necrosis. CBS has been categorized as "threatened," where the carotid artery is exposed to the external environment due to skin breakdown or by direct tumor invasion; "impending," in which a sentinel bleed occur, but is controlled by conservative management; or "acute," where there is active bleeding.

Prior to the advances in endovascular interventions, CBS was managed by open surgical intervention with carotid grafting, ligation, or oversewing. Current management algorithms have shifted away from open surgical treatment if endovascular interventions are available.[3] Patients presenting with acute or impending CBS are hemodynamically stabilized prior to endovascular stenting. Patients with direct carotid artery invasion of tumor or "threatened" CBS can be prophylactically stented. In these circumstances, endovascular procedures have been shown to be effective. If vessels have not yet ruptured, endovascular stents can be used to reinforce the vessel wall. If bleeding has already started, endovascular stents, balloons, or coils may control the bleeding. In any of these scenarios, if tumor is still present, these measures offer mainly a palliative benefit.

REFERENCES

1. Polacare SV, Laing RW, Loomes R. Thorotrast granuloma: an unexpected diagnosis. *J Clin Pathol.* 1992;45:259–261.
2. Wustrow TPU, Behdehani AA, Wiebecke B, Thorotrast induced oro- and hypopharyngeal fibrosis with recurrent bleeding. *J Craniomaxillofac Surg.* 1988;16:315–319.
3. Gaynor BG, Haussen DC, Ambekar S, Peterson EC, Yavagal DR, Elhammady MS. Covered stents for the prevention and treatment of carotid blowout syndrome. *Neurosurgery.* 2015 Aug; 77(2):164–167.

SECTION 6

Professionalism

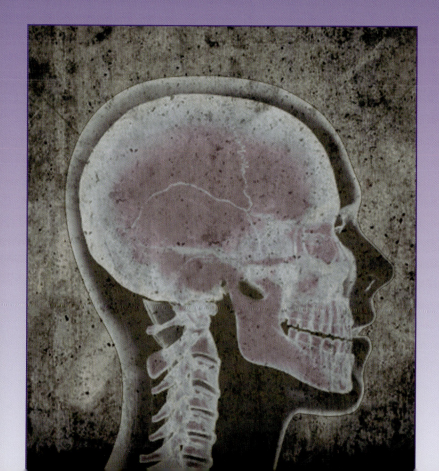

CHAPTER 25

It Was Not Your Fault!

Charles W. Vaughan

In unstable systems, such as human care, even when excellent, "scary" events are normal and to be expected, as are both good and bad outcomes. Although they are to be expected, they cannot be predicted; indeed, many are unknown prior to their appearance.

As an example he cited a case of episodic vertigo (Ménière disease) treated by an attempt at hydrops decompression via opening the endolymphatic sack into the cerebrospinal fluid. However, the intradural location of the sack is often not obvious. I had discovered previously that prior to its entry into the dura the duct could be palpated easily and that following it, it would lead to the sack. This was demonstrated to the resident who was then asked to "try it." On doing so, the resident mumbled, "Oops!" Since how to repair a transected duct was unknown, and since its transection also might provide hydrops relief, the procedure was terminated. On over 6 months follow-up the patient reported no further attacks of vertigo. Wonderful! Great result.

But what about guilt over allowing the transection? Should this have been anticipated? and avoided? Of course—Guilty! But what about the happy, serendipitous discovery of a new therapy? Yes!!! A dumb accident does not deserve praise, but penicillin's discovery resulted in a Nobel Prize. So why not seek some applause? The Swedish report on sham endolymphatic decompression solved this dilemma and further demonstrated that in unstable systems, such as medical care, even when excellent, "scary" events are normal and to be expected, as are both good and bad outcomes. Although they are to be expected, they cannot be predicted; indeed, many are unknown prior to their appearance.

As an afterthought, one other case needs mentioning: debilitating Ménière disease in a farmer from Maine, this time treated with a central nervous system (CNS) vasodilator. On 6-week follow-up, the farmer reported: "I bought the pills on my way home. When I got home and got out of my car, I tripped and spilled my pills all over the yard. The chickens ate 'em . . . and died." [My God! I've killed his chickens!] He stated: "Powerful medicine doc! . . . Haven't had a spell since."

CHARLES W. VAUGHAN (1926–2014)

Dr. Vaughan passed away on March 26, 2014. He was a consummate physician and gifted teacher who continued to teach medical students and residents after his retirement. At the Scary Cases Conference in 2013, Dr. Vaughan made an impromptu lesson on emergency airway techniques in the middle of Dr. Bruce Gordon's presentation of a scary case of anaphylaxis (Figure 25–1).

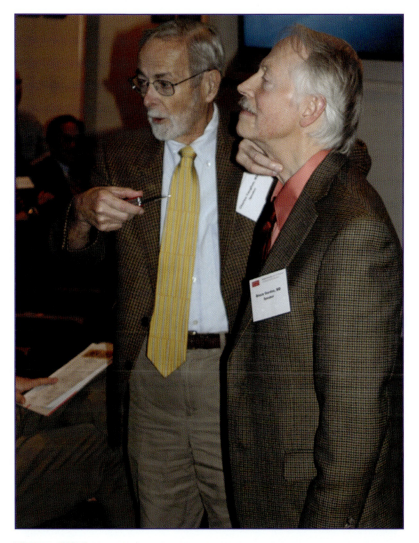

Figure 25–1. Dr. Charles Vaughan teaching emergency airway techniques using a Swiss Army pocket knife to demonstrate cricothyrotomy location on Dr. Bruce Gordon who was presenting a scary case of anaphylaxis.

CHAPTER 26

Tunnel Vision

Too Little . . .
Too Late . . .

Scott Finlay
Mark S. Volk

THE CASE

It was an April night in 1984. I was the PGY-1 surgical resident on call at the Hines VA Hospital, 30 miles west of the Chicago loop. One of my duties as an intern was to help the medicine service gain vascular access on medicine patients on the floor and during emergencies. So the page I answered at around 10:30 PM wasn't that unusual. I had never met the resident who paged me and would never see him again after this encounter. I dialed the call-back number and a voice came on the line. "Mark? Yeah this is Mike Fleming, the PGY-3 on Medicine tonight. We have Mr. Boyer, a 63-year-old man on 9 East, whose pneumonia has taken a turn for the worse and we need to move him up to the unit. But, before we can do that, the ICU nurses said we need to get an art line started. We've been working for about 45 minutes and haven't had any luck. Can you come down and give us a hand?" I agreed to meet him in Mr. Boyer's room in about 5 minutes.

Arterial lines (or "art" lines) are placed within the patient's radial artery as it courses through the wrist. They are commonly used in intensive care settings because they allow continuous blood pressure monitoring and afford the nurses access for blood sampling without disturbing the patient. The line is placed by first feeling for the pulse of the radial artery in the wrist and then cannulating the artery using an IV catheter. While placing these lines can be tricky, most senior medicine residents have mastered this skill, so it must have been at least a little humbling for Mike to call for help from me a PGY-1, 2 years his junior.

I arrived at Mr. Boyer's room on 9 East. As I entered the room I met Mike who was at the bedside along with another Medicine resident, a medical student, and 2 nurses. There were multiple opened and discarded IV catheters on the bed and in the trash. There was something unusual, something going on, that I couldn't put my finger on . . . until later.

Mike filled me in on the patient's situation, "Mr. Boyer's been in the hospital for a couple days on IV antibiotics for his pneumonia. He seemed to be getting better and then a couple hours ago his fever returned and his heart and respiratory rates went up. He might be going into shock. We've been trying to get an art line in before moving him to the unit but Jim (motioning to the other resident) and I've tried multiple times in both arms. I think the artery may be in spasm so we've given it a rest. Maybe you could give it a try?"

Being a resident who was now completing my first (and only!) year of General Surgery, I couldn't imagine that

I wouldn't be able to get the art line in so I approached the task with great enthusiasm. I sat down at the bedside. Mr. Boyer's left wrist had been prepped with antiseptic solution and draped. He was under the cover of a blanket and I couldn't immediately see his face. "OK Mr. Boyer, I'm Dr. Volk and I'm going to try and see if I can place this line in your wrist." There was no reply. I lifted his hand and started to palpate for the radial artery. There were multiple puncture wounds from Mike and Jim's previous attempts. Hmm, it did seem to be in spasm.

After a minute I decided to palpate his left groin in an effort to start at least a temporary art line in the femoral artery. No pulse again. It was then that I looked up at the bedside monitor. The alarms were off, the usual "beeping" sounds associated with the heart rate were absent, and the tracing was flat. Was the monitor not connected? I quickly looked at Mr. Boyer's face. His eyes were open and unseeing with widely, irregularly dilated pupils. A quick palpation of both carotid arteries failed to find a pulse. Mr. Boyer was dead!

And, from the looks of him, he'd been dead for at least a little while. I'm not proud of what happened next. Being near the completion of my General Surgery resident year, I had picked up some of the bravado of my surgical attendings and peers. I say this because that is the only way I can explain what then ensued. "You can't get an art line because he doesn't have a radial pulse and he doesn't have a radial pulse because he's DEAD!," I said in an unkindly way as I looked at the astonished faces of the 5 other caregivers at the bedside and walked out of the room. I remember thinking that they must've all been lazy or incompetent. How else could they have a patient, whom they were actively caring for, die right in front of them and not know it for probably over a half hour?

I never remember seeing any of those doctors and nurses again. But I thought about them and the incident many times over the years. I always wondered how these caregivers could have let this happen? Was this a traumatic experience for them? Did it change their careers, their lives? And, finally, why was my response so callous?

WHAT HAPPENED?

While individuals deliver health care, those individuals almost invariably function as part of a health care team. There are innumerable studies to show that the most common source of errors in medicine is breakdown in team function and communication. The example given above is a result of this type of failure. In the following we discuss the mechanism of error in this particular scenario, the factors that lead up to such errors, the significance of error in medicine, and what we can do to reduce these types of medical errors.

In the described situation, the patient's health care team had identified that he was critically ill and were in the process of arranging for him to be transferred from the floor to the ICU for a more suitable level of care. In making this transfer the team was required to perform two general sets of tasks. The first was completing the necessary steps to make the transfer. These included performing a handoff with the physicians and nurses from the ICU, arranging for transport, notifying the patient's family and the attending physician, writing orders, documenting the patient's condition in the chart, and because the ICU requested it, placing an arterial line. The second set of tasks involved care that every hospitalized patient requires, namely having his or her condition monitored and providing appropriate intervention, if needed.

In the case above, the task at hand, transferring the patient to the ICU, was one the health care team had most likely performed at least several times before. It was not a new or novel task beyond the scope of their current training. So what was different? The group was never debriefed after the incident so it's not possible to know the reasons as to why this happened. But certainly the environment was a possible cause. The setting was likely one of high stress. Possible stressors that may have been present included this particular patient's acuity, the illness level of other patients, or the workload of the health care providers. All of these factors may have caused the team members to actually change their goals. Instead of their main objective being to care for the patient, their primary goal may have shifted to completing their transfer tasks in order to transport the patient to the ICU and thereby reduce the team's clinical workload. But, in the process of affecting the transfer, they concentrated on carrying out the transfer itself and neglected to perform the function of monitoring and managing the patient. They viewed placement of the arterial line as a necessary task to enable them to transfer the patient to the ICU rather than as a tool to be used to improve ongoing, long-term patient monitoring and treatment. This oversight resulted in their missing the diagnosis of patient deterioration and death.

Human error in medicine has received a great deal of attention in recent years as incidents due to human error are now approaching 70% to 80% and even as high as 90%.[1,2] James Reason, PhD, in his studies on understanding human error describes the major elements of production of an error.

These include the nature of the task, the environmental circumstances, the mechanism behind the performance, and the individual.[3] Performance in these situations can be broken down into skill based, rule based, or knowledge based.[4] These three levels extend from unconscious actions all the way to problem solving requiring conscious, effortful analysis of a new situation or above. In terms of the individual, most processing falls into the "schematic control mode," during which time the activity being performed is almost automatic and performed without thought. It is based on previous performance and events that create a model in the brain to follow in the future. In this case, starting out, the residents' performance was most likely operating in a skill-based manner, getting labs, reading vitals, physical exam, etc. However, they must soon transition to addressing the problem itself: how do we better monitor this patient?

> Critical patient + need for hemodynamic monitoring
> = Arterial line.

This is a rule they have created in their mind to treat this exact scenario. In the resident's mind, this must be the answer. The mind would much rather recognize a certain pattern in a new situation and apply a known rule, which is easier and less consuming than creating a new solution. This can lead to overgeneralization of a situation in order to fit a preferred or recognized pattern.[4] But shouldn't we be able to quickly realize things are different this time, or that we need to move on to something else?

As stated above, the environment plays a large role in error production. Multiple conditions have been studied including high workload, inadequate knowledge, stressful situation, boredom, and change. These conditions effect all levels of performance.[2] In the medical field, stress is often a prominent factor in problem-solving scenarios. In these scenarios, information is often coming quickly and changing constantly, and for this reason we see "coning of attention." This concept is where focus is placed on a single piece of information or a single task, often ignoring everything else.[4]

FIXATION

This focus of attention on a single task is similar to the concept of "fixation" in which previous experience alone is used to solve a problem, even to a detriment to the current situation.[5]

The premise behind both of these concepts is that in stressful situations, the time needed to fully evaluate a problem and come up with a novel solution often feels limited. For this reason, we break it into smaller pieces that may be more familiar in an attempt to find a solution we have used before. Once we have a solution we know has worked in the past, we continue to use it even as it continues to fail in the current situation.

The overall clinical picture of the patient above was narrowed to this one task. Multiple unsuccessful attempts are made to achieve the overall goal, using the same technique and the same reasoning. The resident became encompassed by this one problem and was therefore unable to deter from his current path.

When this fails, the resident should slow down and reassess the new problem, however he continues with pattern recognition. This has happened before and during that episode, general surgery was called and the end goal was achieved. When the new resident comes into the picture, although he knows he has a specific goal in mind, he too goes into automatic thinking when he arrives as did the first group of residents, assessing the patient as a whole. It is this return to the big picture that allows him to realize that the patient is actually deceased and, obviously, no longer requires an arterial line.

WHAT I LEARNED FROM THIS CASE

Can fixation and cone of attention be prevented? Studies have been performed to cause and then evaluate fixation with the overall goal of learning how to escape.[5] The key to escape has been both *self-awareness* as well as *advice from an outside source*.[5] Self-awareness requires changing one's habits, which in and of itself is hard enough. Forcing yourself to take breaks when faced with a challenge, allowing at least a minute or two to step away from the task at hand and re-evaluate the entire scenario. Performing these breaks in both normal and complex scenarios will help to make this more of an automatic performance. However, oftentimes the level of focus, especially in a stressful scenario, is too deep, and even our automatic responses disappear as we remain fixated on the problem.

When self-awareness is lost, an outside voice can act as a "voice of reason," to break the detrimental focus and bring back the full reality of the situation. However, as in the scenario above, there were multiple members of the original team who either failed to recognize or were reluctant to communicate to the team the acute change in the patient's status. Was everyone fixated on the art-line? Did anyone notice but not speak up out of fear of repercussion or being ignored?

All of these points show the importance of communication within the team. Everyone should be made to feel comfortable to speak up at anytime to contribute to the team as well as raise any concerns. This alone can help to prevent error as well as break fixation. Additionally, specific roles within the team can help to ensure that although multiple tasks are being performed, the patient as a whole is always being evaluated from a different point of view.

FOLLOW-UP

I wish I could give follow-up of the case, but it ended with me walking out of the room. However, if that same case were to happen today, the ending would have been different. The culture has changed. Quality and safety have moved to the forefront of medicine with continuous efforts to improve care and avoid errors. A root-cause analysis would have been convened to identify the systems errors that led to this unfortunate outcome. Root-cause analyses are commonplace in medicine when there is a catastrophic outcome. All members of the team who were involved in the case would convene in a room with a moderator to discuss all aspects of the case and identify systems errors that led to the problem. As the surgeon finding the mistake, I would have avoided blame or shame with my colleagues, because it is not an individual error that led to the outcome.

PREVENTION

As part of the quality and improvement initiatives that have occurred in medicine over the past 10 years, there has been significant impetus to improve teamwork and communication by adopting teamwork principles. These principles, known as crisis resource management (CRM), have been shown to effectively improve outcomes in enterprises such as the military, aviation, and nuclear power. Teaching such principles involves practice using experiential teaching tools such as medical simulation. Such efforts are showing improvement in teamwork and patient outcomes by changing culture and attitudes.

REFERENCES

1. Reason J. Safety in the operating theatre—part 2: human error and organisational failure. *Qual Saf Health Care*. 2005;14(1):56–60.
2. Reason J. Understanding adverse events: human factors. *Qual Health Care*. 1995;4(2):80–89.
3. Reason J. *Human Error*. Cambridge, UK: Cambridge University Press; 1990.
4. Leape LL. Error in medicine. *JAMA*. 1994;272(23):1851–1857.
5. Fioratou E, Flin R, Glavin R. No simple fix for fixation errors: cognitive processes and their clinical applications. *Anaesthesia*. 2010;65(1):61–69.

CHAPTER 27

Chronic Traumatic Encephalopathy

Who Wants to Fight?

Michael P. Platt

Robert A. Stern

> "I went to a fight and a hockey game broke out."
> —R. Dangerfield

THE CASE

Bob was a 42-year-old ex-professional hockey player who presented to the outpatient Otolaryngology clinic complaining of nasal obstruction and chronic nasal drainage. He suffered from nasal symptoms for as long as he could remember, but he never sought treatment due to other more pressing issues in his life, including a hockey career that spanned his childhood into his mid-30s. He had significant nasal trauma over the years as he was an "enforcer"—a hockey player who was the designated intimidator, instigator, or fighter. The enforcer's role was to fight to change the momentum of the game or intimidate the opponents by fighting or providing hard-hitting that kept opponents off-balance. Professional hockey players generally do not wear protective face masks, resulting in significant facial trauma during fights and "legal" hits.

At our first visit, he wanted to share his life stories. He grew up in a very successful family where his parents and siblings attended prestigious universities. Although he could have "done anything with his life," his parents had focused his energy toward hockey. Over the years, his strength as a hockey player was attributed to his physical game and ability to fight. Unfortunately, he had off-ice mishaps that led to problems with law enforcement and time away from hockey. He was inherently angry that events that were apparently beyond his control had led to a professional career that was far below his potential.

After listening to his story for 20 to 30 minutes, a physical examination revealed a comminuted and deviated nasal septum with nasal polyps in the middle meatii on nasal endoscopy. From a medical standpoint, he had tried numerous nasal medications and systemic therapies, none of which provided significant relief of his sinonasal symptoms. He had a history and physical examination that were consistent with chronic sinusitis with polyps and a septal deviation consistent with fighting on an almost daily basis. He was seeking definitive treatment of his nasal obstruction to improve his quality of life and breathing. He was officially retired from ice hockey, and he thought that his nose would no longer suffer the daily trauma that contributed to his problem.

He returned 2 weeks later following a sinus computed tomography (CT) scan to discuss surgery. He was initially seen by my nurse practitioner, who spent significant time hearing his life story of almost fame and missed glory. She sensed that something was "off" with him, but she could not make a diagnosis. I spent significant time with him to discuss the consent for surgery, and he again told of his life stories and misadventures that limited his ability to "be the best."

Bob clearly had signs of psychosocial abnormalities that were underappreciated in the setting of a specialty surgical clinic. It was my duty as a rhinologist to treat his chronic sinusitis and septal deviation while providing our hospital's motto—"Exceptional Care Without Exception." He agreed to surgery, and a date was selected where his father could bring him for the procedure.

LET THE FIGHT BEGIN

On the morning of surgery, I was alerted by the preoperative nurse that Bob was furious. There had been a cancellation on the night prior, and the nurse had left a voice message on his phone asking if he could come earlier than had been planned. Bob could not understand how a hospital system could change a time at the last minute. I tried to explain the many moving parts of the operating room (OR) schedule—emergencies, cancellations, unexpected delays, etc—but he could not see past the singular event that his OR time was changed without his approval. I offered to cancel or reschedule his surgery, but he angrily chose to proceed. As in the outpatient clinic, the preoperative nurses and anesthesia team commented that something was "off," but there was no clear diagnosis made.

Surgery was uneventful. I was most careful about repairing his septum without injury to the flaps as I sensed that he would not be understanding of a septal perforation. Despite having polyps in the middle meatii, the distal reaches of his sinuses were aerated without signs of inflammation, portending a good prognosis for surgery to alleviate his symptoms of sinusitis. I felt some relief as I completed his surgery without any complication. My relief was short-lived as the case becomes more interested on emergence from anesthesia.

Bob awoke from anesthesia with more anger than I have ever seen. His face was beet red, his stare was unwavering, and he flexed his upper body in intimidation as he requested to fight my 260-pound anesthesiologist who had put him to sleep. There were 5 of us holding Bob on a narrow table as he would not look or listen to anyone else in the room, other than the anesthesiologist whom he was ready to fight. We were scared—especially the anesthesiologist. Perhaps Bob focused on the largest target in the room? The most challenging fight? Or perhaps there was something that the anesthesiologist asked before surgery, that is, "Do you use drugs?" With everyone restraining the patient on a narrow OR table, we asked our anesthesiologist to leave the room as Bob could not stop looking for a fight. Once the anesthesiologist left, Bob refocused his anger.

The next target of our professional "instigator" was the scrub nurse, a 5'8" 170-pound, former minor league hockey player and military veteran. This scrub nurse had seen it all—from working in the military hospitals, VA system, and playing on the hockey circuit—he knew whom he was dealing with. The scrub nurse looked at Bob as just another punk who didn't scare him. The lack of fear fueled Bob's anger and desire for a fight. He was ready to go, until a dose of IV Versed allowed us to safely remove our fighter from the narrow OR table to a stretcher and the recovery room.

The fight was just beginning! Once in the recovery room, Bob decided to tell his perioperative nurse how he felt about nurses: "all nurses are whores," which he followed with additional harassing profanities and verbal threats of physical abuse. As the nurses left the room to call security, I tried to calm him down. He was angry about the way that the nurses looked at him before surgery, as if he were "a second-class citizen." Until this point, he would not acknowledge my presence in the room.

The first safety officer to arrive was confronted by Bob in a similar posture to his emergence from anesthesia—ready for a fight. Five more officers arrived and Bob was ready to take them on, with blood spewing from his mustache dressing from nasal surgery and the IV tubing flailing through the air. It was a scary sight. Bob was still in his stretcher, but as he tried to arise for the big fight, security was required to restrain him as we could not ensure that he was stable for standing following general anesthesia. He was a danger to himself and surely a danger to everyone else with threats of harm and spewing blood. In 5 minutes, the security officers had 4-point restraints in place and Bob was angrier than ever.

What was different about the current anger was that for the first time since he awoke, he looked at me as the target of his rage. I was at his bedside during the previous fights, but he never once acknowledged me as I tried to settle and reassure him. Now that he was in 4-point restraint, he knew that I was the only person who could release him from this situation. "Dr. Platt, How could you do this to me? . . . Is this the way that you treat your patients? . . . This hospital is the worst . . . " As time went on and I didn't give in, his threats became more intense: "Dr. Platt, if you don't release me, I'm going to hurt you . . . I will find you . . . I will find your home . . . I will find your family . . . I will kill you!"

I had to leave the room while the entire recovery area was exposed to an outrageously violent, screaming patient who was saying anything and everything to get a response from passersby. I called his father and informed him of the situation. His father had seen this before and he arrived within a short time, but the fight continued. Bob unleashed a lifetime of insults on his father and his family for not allowing him to reach his potential. As time went on, Bob's father was able to reason with him that if he didn't stop, he would be admitted to a psychiatric ward for safety. The threat of long-term restraint was enough to get Bob to internalize his anger, although everyone could sense his desire to fight.

WHAT NEXT?

Can you release a patient following surgery who has not met the usual criteria and stops of recovery? The anesthesiologist was not comfortable releasing the restraints in the recovery area, or taking the responsibility that the patient had adequately recovered from anesthesia. Bob was transferred to the emergency department (ED) via stretcher with 4-point restraints in place. He had a harassing comment for each person who looked at him on the journey across the hospital.

The ED physician knew what to do. After he introduced himself to Bob, he asked Bob "What's going on?" Bob replied, "I bet you live in F . . . ing Wellesley (an upscale suburb of Boston)." The ED physician replied, "You are free to go." I was shocked, but it worked—Bob immediately relented. The safety officers removed the restraints, I gave Bob his postoperative instructions, and he stood up, shook hands with every security officer, and said, "Thanks so much, Good job!" Bob congratulated each member of the team as if we just had a hockey fight and the game was over.

THE CLEAN-UP

Now what? I just did surgery on someone who threatened to find my home and kill me and my family. Was he serious? Can you ignore such a threat? What about the follow-up? He needs to have septal splints removed and sinuses débrided on the following week. I felt bad for exposing my staff to risk and harassment. Should I have known beforehand? Could I possibly bring him back and expose my office staff to a patient with such anger and threats? And my family? That evening, I Googled my name and found my address within 1 minute on the Internet. Was my family in danger?

Needless to say, it was a long week of poor sleep and phone calls. My first call was to my Chairman, Dr. Ken Grundfast, to let him know what happened. Ken is always supportive, especially in times of trouble. He suggested that I contact Patient Advocacy, who provides support when there are disputes between patients and staff. The patient advocate listened to my story and suggested that I release the patient from Boston Medical Center. There are clear steps that can be instituted when firing a patient, but one of the essential components —finding appropriate follow-up—was not an option. We are fortunate to have an extremely collegial group of Otolaryngologists in Boston, all of whom I respect and like. There was no way I could displace the risks and dangers of this patient's follow-up visit on a colleague I respected.

Now that I recognized that I had to see him and débride his sinuses, I needed a plan for getting him through my clinic without an incident. Safety was my primary concern, so I called an educator from the public safety department. He patiently listened to the story and advised that I call Bob and his father to get a sense of the risk, and then if acceptable, I should see him alone in the clinic. He advised that this personality would be more stable without a safety officer or advocate present, which could instigate a fight. He recommended that the safety officers be in the vicinity during the visit, but otherwise treat it as a regularly scheduled follow-up, minus the usual wait-time as Bob does not do well with changes in the schedule.

I called Bob's primary care physician who only met him once and could not provide additional insight to help the situation. I then spoke to his father who conveyed Bob's troubled past and difficulties with authority. He reassured me that Bob was "all talk" and not a true threat to anyone. I called Bob, who wanted to know why I restrained him "for no reason." He claimed to have no recollection of the events leading up to the restraint. After explaining the situation, he apologized, and I made plans for his postoperative follow-up a few days later.

The follow-up visit occurred without incident, as if there were never a fight in the OR. I removed the splint and suctioned old blood and mucous from his sinuses. I encouraged Bob to seek counseling for underlying problems with anger and instability, but Bob had already "been through" all of those, "many times" without help. I was relieved that he had the surgical outcomes that I had hoped for without any difficulties, but I knew that something bad would happen eventually with his underlying problems.

I thought that I would not hear from Bob again, having performed an apparent successful surgery and having gone through a traumatic ordeal for all of the parties involved. However, I received a phone call from him 2 months later. I returned his call and he had a problem. His brother punched him in the face ("for no reason") and caused a nasal deformity. He asked if I could fix his nose. Upholding the motto of Boston Medical Center, I agreed to see him within a few days. I performed a closed reduction of a nasal fracture under local anesthesia in my office. There was no chance that I could expose him—and my OR staff—to general anesthesia again.

THE DIAGNOSIS

Chronic traumatic encephalopathy (CTE) is a neurodegenerative disease that is caused by repetitive head trauma.[1-3] Bob was a fighter. He made a career in professional hockey by his aggressive play, legal checking (hitting), and fist fighting, both on and off the ice. Head trauma was a daily occurrence for Bob, and it resulted in loss of brain function. Bob had problems with mood, behavior, and cognition, which are hallmarks of CTE.

CTE was initially described in boxers who displayed a "punch drunk" personality, but later had mental deterioration that sometimes resulted in commitment to an asylum. It is well documented that boxers have suffered from both mood and behavior problems later in life. Repetitive head injuries can lead to motor symptoms and frank dementia in severe cases, although it is unknown if certain patterns or mechanisms of trauma lead to specific impairments. An early published description of the behavior changes in CTE, describing "disinhibition, irritability, hypomania, impaired insight, paranoia, and violent outbursts"[4] are eerily consistent with Bob's personality.

Head trauma is a necessary requirement for the development of CTE, but not all people with repetitive head trauma will develop CTE. The incidence and prevalence of CTE remain unknown because there is no accepted and accurate method of diagnosing CTE during life. The diagnosis of CTE is usually made on postmortem autopsies of individuals who have had repetitive head trauma. Pathologic findings include accumulation of a hyperphosphorylated tau protein in a pattern specific to CTE.[1-3] Accumulation of tau protein begins in the cortex, and then spreads more medially in advancing stages of the disease. This is in contrast to Alzheimer disease, where tau pathology first occurs in the brainstem and spreads to the cortex.

The clinical features of CTE can be classified as cognitive, behavioral, mood, and motor.[1-3] Younger patients often suffer from behavior and mood disturbances, whereas old patients demonstrate cognitive features of CTE with impairment in memory, executive function, attention, lack of insight, language, and/or dementia. Behavioral problems in CTE include violence, explosivity, loss of control, paranoia, aggression, boastfulness, disinhibited behavior, personality changes, and psychosis. Mood disturbances include depression, anxiety, irritability, labile emotions, mania, and mood swings. The motor features of CTE are demonstrated by the famous boxer Muhammad Ali, who suffered from ataxia, dysarthria, parkinsonism features, tremor, masked facies, rigidity, and weakness.

CTE is a progressive disease with no known cure and limited treatment options for managing symptoms (Table 27–2). Counseling is often provided for the mood and behavioral problems; however, the loss of cognition and insight often makes it difficult for patients to understand their disorder and accept treatment. For patients with CTE, management strategies to avoid the situation encountered in Bob's case include a calming environment with frequent reassurance, regular physical and cognitive exercises, and daily rituals that provide a stable environment. Bob's experience in the operating room provided a new environment with a changing schedule, unfa-

Table 27–1. Steps to Releasing a Patient From Your Practice

1. Document reasons for dismissal from the practice.
2. Ensure that emergency treatment is not needed.
3. Provide written notification via certified mail including reasons for termination.
4. Provide a listing of other providers who can assume care.

miliar faces, the stress of surgery, and anesthetic medications that removed inhibitions, which all provided an unfavorable setting that triggered Bob's outburst.

Bob's case is sad because all of his mood, behavioral, and cognitive problems can be attributed to CTE. Bob was a child prodigy—cultivated by his family to achieve greatness in a sport with deep roots in New England. He was a product of early morning skates, weekend trips to tournaments, and daily training that resulted in a lifetime of head trauma on the ice. Now in his 40s, Bob has a scary future. He has difficulty maintaining employment, keeping relationships with his family, and navigating the world without hockey. With no known cure or successful treatment for CTE, avoidance of head trauma in sports is essential in preventing the development of CTE.

THIS CASE WAS SCARY BECAUSE

This case was scary because I was placed at personal risk by a patient who threatened to kill me and my family. I also placed my staff at risk for injury and as a target of verbal abuse. It was scary that I had no way out, because I could not refer him to a colleague who would be at the same risk as me. Finally, CTE is a scary diagnosis because there is no good treatment option or cure. Patients are often a risk to themselves with a high number of suicides associated with chronic depression, substance abuse, and lack of treatment.

WHAT I LEARNED FROM THIS CASE

1. Don't ever feel compelled to treat someone whom you are not comfortable treating. As a physician and surgeon, you decide whom to operate on and whom to treat. You do not need to care for patients whom you do not share a safe, professional relationship (Table 27–1).

Table 27–2. Care of Patients With Chronic Traumatic Encephalopathy
Counseling for the mood and behavioral problems
Calming environment
Frequent reassurance
Regular physical and cognitive exercises
Daily rituals that provide a stable environment

There are always other clinicians who may be able to have such a relationship with patients who have particular personalities or confounding disorders.
2. Having the correct diagnosis and the option for surgery are only part of what is needed to pursue a surgery for a "quality-of-life" indication. Patients need to have the insight and appropriate behavior that will allow them to consent, prepare, and recover from surgery. Performing the actual surgery is often "easier" than the pre-op and post-op care that is needed to achieve successful outcomes.
3. Always ask for help when you get in a difficult situation. The ED physician, my chairman, the patient advocate, and the safety officer provided essential advice in resolving this conflict without incident.
4. Chronic traumatic encephalopathy is a very sad and difficult disease because it is usually avoidable, essentially untreatable, and often results in a poor prognosis.

ASK THE EXPERT: Anthony Abeln, JD

When and how do you release a patient from your practice?

Releasing a patient from your practice is certainly one of the least pleasant experiences any physician can face. By no means does a physician need to expose himself or herself, or a practice staff, to physical, psychological, or emotional harm. Moreover, where a patient reasonably presents an immediate threat to a physician or physician's family, as here, it is entirely appropriate for a physician to involve law enforcement. That said, however, the Emergency Medical Treatment and Active Labor Act (EMTALA) can present some threshold challenges. Is the violent or threatening behavior itself part of a behavioral, psychiatric, or other medical condition? Further, if the patient requires emergency care, generally, that care must be provided.

In the absence of any emergency situation, and to avoid any appearance of patient abandonment, termination of the patient from your practice needs to be a well-documented and thorough process. The patient needs to be provided adequate notice to obtain treatment from another provider and be offered bridge care until that transition has occurred. The notice should also describe in detail the reasons why the doctor has chosen to terminate the patient. Your office should be prepared to assist with transitioning the patient to a new provider. While these situations almost always turn on fact-specific circumstances, a well-documented procedure in notifying the patient that you will no longer be able to assist, along with extensive notice can assist in avoiding a complaint.

REFERENCES

1. Montenigro PH, Corp DT, Stein TD, Cantu RC, Stern RA. Chronic traumatic encephalopathy: historical origins and current perspective. *Annu Rev Clin Psychol*. 2015;11:309–330.
2. Montenigro PH, Baugh CM, Daneshvar DH, et al. Clinical subtypes of chronic traumatic encephalopathy: literature review and proposed research diagnostic criteria for traumatic encephalopathy syndrome. *Alzheimer Res Ther*. 2014 Sep 24;6(5):68.
3. Stern RA, Daneshvar DH, Baugh CM, et al. Clinical presentation of chronic traumatic encephalopathy. *Neurology*. 2013 Sep 24; 81(13):1122–1129.
4. Jordan BD. Chronic traumatic brain injury associated with boxing. *Semin Neurol*. 2000;20(2):179–185.

CHAPTER 28

Helping Your Colleague

No Good Deed Goes Unpunished

Aaron R. Dezube
Christopher W. Tsang
Mark Vecchiotti

THE CASE

A 2½-year-old girl, with no significant past medical history other than being born at 36 weeks' gestation, was seen in the pediatric otolaryngology clinic for snoring and found to have adenotonsillar hypertrophy. Her history and physical exam findings were consistent with obstructive sleep apnea (OSA), and she was recommended to undergo adenotonsillectomy for relief of her symptoms. Her parents, both of whom were employees at the hospital (mother is a pediatric intensive care unit [PICU] nurse and father is a respiratory therapist), agreed to the procedure, and she was scheduled for surgery.

On the day of surgery, the primary surgeon developed severe vertigo and was unable to come to the hospital. The primary surgeon asked his colleague to perform the surgery both as a favor to him and to the patient's family. Knowing the family as professional colleagues, both the patient's parents and I agreed to this change. In the preoperative area the patient was noted to have had 2 episodes of tonsillitis (both times positive for group A β-hemolytic streptococcus) since her last clinic visit. She had just finished a 10-day course of amoxicillin 2 days prior to surgery, and was asymptomatic. Her preoperative exam was unremarkable, without any tonsillar or pharyngeal inflammation, and she was also cleared for surgery by pediatric anesthesia.

I performed the procedure myself, with a PGY-3 resident present as first assist. The tonsils were removed in an extracapsular fashion using monopolar cautery on a setting of 20 watts, and the adenoids were removed with suction cautery on a setting of 28 watts. There was little to no need for hemostasis in the tonsillar fossae. Incidentally, we noted a small 1 to 2-mm dehiscence of the constrictor muscle in the mid-tonsillar fossa on the left, through which a small bleb of parapharyngeal fat could be visualized. At the time, both the resident and I agreed that the defect was likely congenital rather than iatrogenic, as no muscle tissue was violated during the case and the use of cautery for hemostasis was minimal. Given the small size of the defect, we decided to allow it to heal via secondary intention, rather than suturing it closed.

During extubation, the patient experienced some moderate laryngospasm requiring positive pressure bag-mask ventilation, but did not need to be re-intubated. However, as a result of the laryngospasm episode, we decided to admit the patient to the PICU, instead of her planned admission to the regular hospital floor, postoperatively (Figure 28–1). The patient's

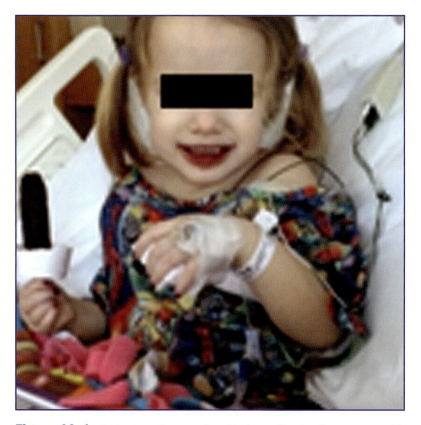

Figure 28-1. Patient resting comfortably immediately after surgery with no neck cellulitis.

recovery was unremarkable until approximately 12 hours after the procedure, at which point she had several bouts of emesis. Shortly after this, she developed progressive swelling of her neck and face and a persistent fever (Figure 28-2). The following morning, her neck swelling continued to worsen, and she developed tachycardia and hypotension in addition to the fever. She required multiple intravenous fluid boluses and was started on broad-spectrum antibiotics (vancomycin, piperacillin/tazobactam, and clindamycin).

Blood cultures were obtained, and initial laboratory tests were significant for a white blood cell count of 15.6 and a C-reactive protein (CRP) level of 131.65. A computed tomography (CT) scan of the neck with contrast demonstrated air in the parapharyngeal space that had tracked inferiorly to the hypopharynx and crossed the midline (Figure 28-3). This constellation of findings was consistent with sepsis secondary to necrotizing fasciitis.

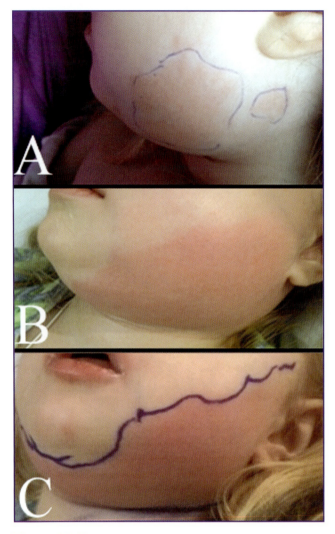

Figure 28–2. Progression of cellulitis to necrotizing fasciitis at 8 hours postoperatively (**A**), 20 hours postoperatively (**B**), and 24 hours postoperatively (**C**).

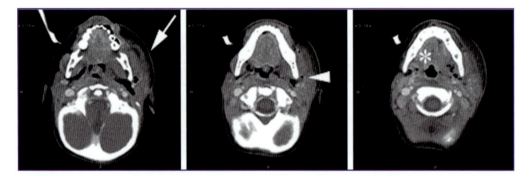

Figure 28–3. Axial CT scan of the neck demonstrating air in the parapharyngeal space lateral to angle of the mandible (*arrowhead*), extending inferiorly with associated left facial swelling (*arrow*), and tracking across midline at the level of the hypopharynx (*asterisk*).

In front of a growing audience consisting of the patient's family, the other's coworkers in the PICU, the on-call PICU attending and his colleagues, and residents from various services who happened to be present, the parents were informed of the need for an emergency surgical procedure, to which they readily agreed. Unfortunately, as the patient was being rushed to the surgical suite, I was performing a complex tympanomastoidectomy with ossicular chain reconstruction with a PGY-4 resident who had never performed the procedure before. We quickly called one of our head and neck surgeons from clinic (in the same building) to assist in getting the patient to the operating room and to help establish the airway if necessary. Fortunately, I was able to finish the critical aspects of my otologic case and run into this patient's room just as she was arriving. There, I found not just my head and neck surgery colleague, but the entire otolaryngology department, waiting in the room to watch, and assist if necessary. The patient was stable on arrival to the operating room and was intubated without issue.

The left parapharyngeal space was accessed transorally through the tonsillar fossa, and extensive débridement was performed of necrotic tissue, including fat and portions of the constrictor muscle. No frank purulence was encountered, although there was an abundance of seropurulent "dishwater" fluid within the tissue planes. There was no evidence of any extension to the carotid sheath. The wound was thoroughly irrigated out with antibiotic solution, and the patient was returned to the PICU intubated.

What happened was a potentially life-threatening postoperative complication from an otherwise routine surgery. In retrospect, this patient had an anatomic dehiscence that provided a direct pathway to the parapharyngeal space, and she was likely still colonized with group A β-hemolytic streptococcus. Postoperatively, the patient had laryngospasm requiring positive pressure ventilation and subsequent emesis, both likely widening this dehiscence, and seeding the parapharyngeal space. The overall result was the development of postoperative cervical necrotizing fasciitis requiring emergecy débridement.

THIS CASE WAS SCARY BECAUSE

This was scary for several reasons:

1. The development of a rapidly progressing and potentially fatal complication on a completely healthy young girl as a result of a fairly routine procedure

2. Assuming care of another surgeon's patient on the day of a planned elective procedure
3. My personal relationship with the patient's family
4. The fact that the patient's parents were care providers at the hospital where this complication occurred (in fact, the mother worked in the PICU where the majority of this patient's care took place)
5. My initial unavailability to manage an emergent complication from a procedure that I performed, and the need for further intraoperative cross-coverage by another one of my colleagues
6. The conflicting motivation for wanting to be the one to take care of my complication while actively engaged in a complex procedure on another patient
7. The perceived (but certainly not real) scrutiny when managing a complication such as this in front of my department and professional colleagues as well as the professional colleagues of the patient's parents

WHAT I LEARNED FROM THIS CASE

What I learned from this case is the following:

1. To be prepared for uncommon and rare complications of common procedures
2. To be aware of the risks you may be assuming when you take over a patient who is not "yours"
3. To know when to call for help from colleagues, despite the strong personal feelings of responsibility and need to manage one's own complications, and furthermore, not to let these feelings jeopardize the care of one patient for another
4. To use clear and unbiased medical judgment in the face of multiple extrinsic professional and social stressors in a rapidly developing situation

REVIEW OF THE LITERATURE

Necrotizing fasciitis is an aggressive bacterial infection that spreads across fascial planes, with rapid involvement of adjacent tissue. While necrotizing fasciitis is a severe and potentially fatal soft tissue infection, involvement of the head and neck is rare with only a handful of cases caused by tonsillitis or peritonsillar abscesses described in the literature. These few reported cases were primarily caused by a streptococcal bacterial subtype.[1,2] The etiology is likely explained by the fact that most cases of bacterial tonsillitis are due to group A β-hemolytic streptococcus. Tonsillar necrotizing fasciitis has the potential to develop into cervical necrotizing fasciitis, which has a poor prognosis and may lead to mediastinitis and septic shock.[3,4] Often, necrotizing fasciitis of the head and neck leads to permanent disfigurement as it involves the skin, subcutaneous tissue, adjacent tissue, and muscles quickly, and requires aggressive medical and surgical intervention.[5] Computed tomography scans may show characteristic patterns allowing early recognition of necrotizing fasciitis, such diffuse enhancement and thickening of the platysma, strap muscles, and sternocleidomastoid, as well as fluid in multiple compartments of the neck.[6]

It is interesting to note that at this time, there does not seem to be any literature to date regarding the risks or outcomes of surgery performed by cross-covering physicians.

CASE OUTCOME

Postoperatively, the patient was extubated immediately and recovered quickly. Although penicillin-sensitive group A β-hemolytic streptococcus was found on blood cultures, the intraoperative wound cultures were all negative for any bacterial growth. The patient was transitioned to monotherapy with ceftriaxone and was discharged home on postoperative day 6. The patient has since been seen in clinic several times without any further complications, and is currently happy and healthy.

REFERENCES

1. Zilberstein B, De Cleva R, Testa RS, Sene U, Eshkenazy R, Gama-Rodrigues JJ. Cervical necrotizing fasciitis due to bacterial tonsillitis. *Clinics (Sao Paulo)*. 2005;60(2):177–182.
2. Skitarelić N, Mladina M, Morović M, Skitarelić N. Cervical necrotizing fasciitis: sources and outcomes. *Infection*. 2003;31(1):39–44.
3. Mathieu D, Neviere R, Teillon C, Chagnon JL, Lebleu N, Wattel F. Cervical necrotizing fasciitis: clinical manifestations and management. *Clin Infect Dis*. 1995;21:51–56.
4. Islam A, Oko M. Cervical necrotizing fasciitis and descending mediastinitis secondary to unilateral tonsillitis: a case report. *J Med Case Rep*. 2008;2:368.

5. Klabacha ME, Stankiewicz JA, Clift SE. Severe soft tissue infection of the face and neck: a classification. *Laryngoscope*. 1982;92:1135–1139.
6. Becker M, Zbären P, Hermans R, et al. Necrotizing fasciitis of the head and neck: role of computed tomography in diagnosis and management. *Radiology*. 1997;202:471–476.